CARNIVORE DIET 2025

120 Recipes Weight Loss and Wellbeing With the Power of Meat Meal Plan to Optimize Your Wellbeing

KLARLOCK

DISCLAIMER

This book aims to provide useful and informative material on the topics covered in the publication. It is sold with the understanding that the author and publisher are not engaged in rendering any personal medical, health care, or other professional services in the book. The reader should consult his or her physician, health care provider, or other competent professional before adopting any suggestions in this book or drawing any conclusions. The author and publisher expressly disclaim any responsibility for any liability, loss, or risk, personal or otherwise, arising, directly or indirectly, from the use and application of any contents of this book.

NOTE

All the recipes in this book are designed for four people. For this quantity, the ingredients indicated in the recipes must be considered. If you need to change the portion, it is recommended to proportionally adjust the doses of the ingredients. It is also recommended to carefully follow the preparation and cooking instructions to obtain the best result. In the context of this book, when we refer to "a cup" as a unit of measurement for ingredients, we mean using a standard kitchen cup with a capacity of approximately 240 milliliters. It is essential to use a measuring cup to get the right quantities of ingredients. If you don't have a measuring cup, you can use a graduated measuring cup, making sure to correctly correspond to the proportions indicated. Here are some examples 1 Cup of flour 100 gr. 1 cup of rice 200 gr. 1 Cup of Quinoa 200 gr

TABLE OF CONTENT

RECIPES FIRST DISHES

150 TOMATO SOUP WITH CRISPY HAM

152 CHICKEN AND VEGETABLE LASAGNE

155 PILOT RICE WITH SAUSAGE

157 LINGUINE WITH CLAMS AND BACON

159 SORRENTINA GNOCCHI WITH COOKED HAM

161 BLACK BEAN SOUP WITH CHORIZO

163 RISOTTO WITH PORCINI MUSHROOMS

166 FUSILLI WITH MEAT SAUCE

168 TORTELLINI WITH BACON AND CREAM

170 PAPPARDELLE WITH RABBIT SAUCE

172 CHICKEN SOUP WITH VEGETABLES AND COUSCOUS

174 TAGLIATELLE WITH LAMB SAUCE

176 PASTA AND BEANS WITH BACON

178 HAM AND CHEESE RAVIOLI WITH BUTTER AND SAGE

RECIPES SECOND DISHES

206 BEEF BURGER WITH MELTED CHEESE

208 GRILLED TUNA STEAK

210 CHICKEN STUFFED WITH HAM AND CHEESE

213 GRILLED MIXED MEAT SKEWERS

215 BEEF FILLET WITH GREEN PEPPER SAUCE

217 CHICKEN CACCIATORA

219 LAMB CHOPS WITH ROSEMARY

221 HORSE STEAK WITH GARLIC SAUCE

223 ROAST PORK WITH BAKED POTATOES

225 VENETIAN-STYLE VEAL LIVER

227 BEEF CHOP WITH TOMATO SAUCE

230 PORK SAUSAGES WITH MASHED POTATOES

232 BARBECUE LAMB RIBS

234 GRILLED DUCK STEAK

236 CHICKEN WITH LEMON AND PARSLEY

INTRODUCTION TO THE CARNIVORE DIET

The carnivore diet is a diet that involves the exclusive consumption of products of animal origin, completely excluding plant foods such as fruit, vegetables, cereals and legumes. This diet has become popular in recent years thanks to media attention and the stories of people who have benefited from it for their health. Fundamentals of the Carnivore Diet The carnivorous diet is based on the idea that human beings are biologically predisposed to eat mainly meat and animal products. Proponents of this diet believe that a diet rich in animal proteins and healthy fats is optimal for health and can help prevent and manage a number of health conditions, such as inflammation, digestive problems, and metabolic disorders.

Recommended Foods In the carnivore diet, the main foods are: Red meat: beef, lamb, pork, game. Poultry: chicken, turkey. Eggs: A versatile source of protein. Animal fats: butter, lard, lard. Offal: liver, heart, kidneys, which are particularly nutritious. Benefits and Criticisms Supporters say the carnivore diet can improve mental and physical health, reduce inflammation and promote weight loss. However, there are also criticisms and concerns related to this regimen, mainly regarding the lack of fiber, essential vitamins and minerals present in vegetables, and the potential negative effects on the cardiovascular system. Advice and Precautions Before embarking on the carnivorous diet, it is important to consult a health professional, especially to evaluate any risks to your specific health. Additionally, it is recommended to carefully monitor nutrient levels and supplement with vitamins and minerals as needed.

WHAT IS THE CARNIVORE DIET

The carnivore diet is a diet that involves the exclusive consumption of foods of animal origin, completely eliminating vegetables. This means that those who follow this diet eat only meat, fish, eggs and dairy products, excluding fruit, vegetables, cereals, legumes and other plant foods. Basic Principles The philosophy behind the carnivore diet is based on the idea that humans evolved as carnivores or at least as predominantly meat eaters, and that many modern health problems arise from a diet that includes too many carbohydrates and plants. Proponents of the carnivore diet say that a diet rich in animal proteins and fats is more natural for the human body and can lead to improvements in mental and physical health. Permitted Foods Red Meats: such as beef, pork, lamb and game. White Meat: such as chicken and turkey. Fish and Seafood: including salmon, tuna, crustaceans and molluscs.

Eggs: any type. Dairy products: such as butter, cheese, and yogurt (if tolerated). Offal: such as liver, heart and kidneys. Exclusions The carnivore diet completely excludes all plant-based foods, including: Fruits and vegetables Legumes Grains and grain products Nuts and seeds Benefits and Potential Risks Some advocates say this diet can help you lose weight, improve mental health, reduce inflammation and relieve the symptoms of some chronic diseases. However, there are also concerns about potential risks, such as deficiencies of essential nutrients (for example, fiber, vitamins and minerals found in plants) and long-term effects on cardiovascular health. Considerations As with any diet, it is important to carefully consider your health goals and, if possible, consult a health professional before starting a new diet. The carnivore diet is particularly restrictive and may not be suitable for everyone.

ORIGINS AND HISTORY OF THE CARNIVORE DIET

The carnivore diet is one of the oldest diets, dating back to the times when humans lived as hunter-gatherers. Throughout most of human history, populations fed primarily on meat and fish, as plant resources were seasonal and often limited. This style of eating was typical of populations living in cold climates, where hunting and fishing were the main sources of food. In recent decades, the carnivore diet has been rediscovered and promoted by some health professionals and athletes who claim that a meat-only diet can improve health and physical performance. Modern interest in this diet is often attributed to individuals such as Dr. Shawn Baker, an orthopedic surgeon and athlete who popularized the diet through social media and various podcasts, and to Jordan Peterson, a well-known clinical psychologist who, along with her daughter Mikhaila Peterson, spoke about the benefits she experienced from adopting a carnivorous diet. Fundamental Principles of the Carnivore Diet 1. Exclusive Consumption of Animal Foods: The diet is based on the intake of meat, fish, eggs and, in some cases, dairy products. The consumption of plant foods, including fruits, vegetables, grains, legumes, nuts and seeds, is completely avoided. 2. High Intake of Proteins and Fats: The diet is naturally rich in proteins and fats, which constitute the main source of energy. Particular attention is paid to the intake of saturated fats, present in abundance in products of animal origin. 3. Zero Carbohydrate Reduction: By completely eliminating plant foods, the carnivore diet reduces carbohydrate intake to negligible levels. This can put the body into a state of ketosis, where fat is used as the main source of energy. 4. Simplicity and Satiety: One of the declared advantages of the carnivore diet is its simplicity. Since the number of foods allowed is limited, food decisions become easier. Additionally, protein and fat tend to be very filling, which can help reduce your overall calorie intake without feeling hungry. 5. Elimination of Potential Antinutrients: Proponents of the carnivorous diet argue that many plants contain antinutrients such as lectins, phytates, and oxalates, which can interfere with nutrient absorption and cause digestive or autoimmune problems. By eliminating the plants, these potential problems would be avoided. Considerations and Precautions The carnivorous diet is extremely restrictive and can pose risks of nutritional deficiencies, especially fiber, vitamins and minerals found mainly in plant foods. Therefore, it is essential to consult a doctor or nutritionist before embarking on this diet, and carefully monitor your health during it.

MACRONUTRIENTS IN THE CARNIVORE DIET

The carnivore diet is unique in that it eliminates all carbohydrates and relies exclusively on proteins and fats derived from animal sources. Let's see how macronutrients are distributed in this diet. 1. Protein Protein is a central component of the carnivore diet and comes mainly from meat, fish, eggs and dairy products. These proteins provide all the essential amino acids needed for building and repairing tissue, maintaining muscle mass and supporting the immune system. 2. Fats Fats make up a significant portion of calorie intake in the carnivore diet. These include saturated and unsaturated fats from meat (such as beef, pork, lamb), fatty fish (such as salmon and tuna), butter, lard, and other sources of animal fat. Fats provide energy, aid in the absorption of fat-soluble vitamins (A, D, E, K) and contribute to hormone production. 3. Carbohydrates In the carnivorous diet, carbohydrates are practically absent, since all plant foods are excluded. This often leads to a significant reduction in insulin and can induce a state of ketosis, where the body uses fat as its main energy source. Micronutrients in the Carnivorous Diet Although the carnivorous diet can provide some micronutrients, the absence of plant foods raises concerns about potential deficiencies in some essential nutrients. 1. Vitamins Vitamin B12: Essential for nervous function and the formation of red blood cells, it is abundant in products of animal origin. Vitamin A: In the form of retinol, it is found in the liver and other organs. Vitamin D: Can be obtained from fatty fish and liver, but sun exposure remains an important source. Group B vitamins: Present in meat, especially offal. 2. Minerals Iron: Heme, the most easily absorbable form of iron, is abundant in red meats and offal. Zinc: Essential for immune function and protein synthesis, it is present in many meats. Selenium: Found in meats, fish and eggs, and is important for thyroid function and antioxidant protection. Calcium: May be more limited on a carnivorous diet, especially if you don't consume dairy. Animal bones may be a source, but in general, calcium intake may be low. 3. Fiber and Antioxidants Dietary fibre, essential for intestinal health and cholesterol regulation, is absent in the carnivorous diet, as it is only present in plant foods. Antioxidants, which help protect cells from oxidative damage, are also less present than in a more balanced diet that includes fruit and vegetables. Final Thoughts While providing high quality proteins and fats, the carnivorous diet can lead to deficiencies of some nutrients if not carefully monitored.

BENEFITS OF THE CARNIVORE DIET

Weight Loss One of the main reasons many people choose to follow the carnivore diet is weight loss. This result can be attributed to several factors intrinsic to the diet: 1. Reduction of Carbohydrates The carnivorous diet completely eliminates carbohydrates, including sugars, cereals and starchy vegetables. Reducing carbohydrates often causes the body to enter a state of ketosis, in which it uses fats, including stored fats, as its main source of energy. This process can accelerate body fat loss. 2. Greater Satiety Proteins and fats, which form the basis of the carnivorous diet, are known to induce a longer-lasting feeling of satiety than carbohydrates. This means that people tend to eat less frequently and in smaller quantities, reducing their overall calorie intake without feeling hungry.

3. Stabilizing Blood Sugar Levels
Eliminating carbohydrates can help stabilize blood sugar levels and reduce insulin spikes. This is especially beneficial for people with insulin resistance or type 2 diabetes, as it reduces levels of insulin, a hormone that promotes fat storage. 4. Thermogenic Effect of Proteins Proteins have a higher thermogenic effect than carbohydrates and fats, which means that the body burns more calories to digest proteins. This increase in energy expenditure may further contribute to weight loss. 5. Elimination of Processed Foods By following a carnivorous diet, you completely avoid processed foods, which often contain added sugars, unhealthy oils and artificial ingredients. The elimination of these foods contributes to an overall reduction in calories and an improvement in nutritional quality. 6. Improved Body Composition

The carnivore diet can help maintain or increase muscle mass due to the high protein content. This is important because muscles are metabolically active and help burn calories even at rest, thus improving body composition. 7. Better Appetite Control The combination of proteins and fats, in addition to stabilizing blood sugars, can contribute to better appetite control. This can help people avoid unnecessary snacking and maintain a calorie deficit, which is necessary for weight loss. Final Thoughts Although the carnivore diet can be effective for weight loss, it is important to remember that each person is unique and may respond differently to this diet. Furthermore, sustainable weight loss and long-term health should always be the priority, so it is advisable to consult a health professional before starting the diet.

RECIPES APPETIZERS

BEEF CARPACCIO WITH ARUGULA AND OF PARMESAN FLAKES

doses for 4 people

Ingredients

400 g quality beef (preferably fillet)

100 g of fresh Arugula

50 g of parmesan flakes

Juice of 1 lemon

Extra virgin olive oil

Salt and freshly ground black pepper

Preparation:

Place the beef in the freezer for about 3040 minutes, to make it easier to slice. In the meantime, wash and dry the rocket well. Take the beef from the freezer and slice it as thinly as possible with a sharp knife. Arrange the slices of meat in an even layer on a serving platter. Season the meat with lemon juice, extra virgin olive oil, salt and freshly ground black pepper. Sprinkle the arugula over the beef. Add the parmesan flakes on top of the carpaccio. Serve immediately as a starter or light main course.

RAW HAM AND MELON

doses for 4 people

Ingredients:

200 g of raw ham

1 ripe melon

Fresh mint leaves (optional)

Preparation:

Cut the melon in half, remove the seeds and cut the pulp into slices or cubes, depending on your preference. Arrange the raw ham on a serving plate. Accompany the ham with slices or cubes of melon. If you wish, you can garnish the dish with some fresh mint leaves to add a touch of freshness. Serve as an appetizer or as part of a summer buffet.

TUNA TARTARE WITH AVOCADO

Ingredients:

doses for 4 people

300 g of high quality fresh tuna

1 ripe avocado

Juice of 1 lemon

Extra virgin olive oil

Salt and freshly ground black pepper

Toasted sesame seeds (optional)

Chopped fresh chives or parsley (optional)

Preparation:

Cut the tuna into very small cubes and place it in a bowl. Peel and finely chop the avocado, then add it to the tuna. Squeeze lemon juice onto the tuna and avocado mixture to prevent the avocado from oxidizing and to add a touch of freshness. Season with extra virgin olive oil, salt and freshly ground black pepper. Stir gently to combine the ingredients. If desired, you can add toasted sesame seeds for a crunch or chopped fresh chives or parsley for an additional pop of color and flavor. Cover the bowl with cling film and leave to rest in the fridge for about 30 minutes to allow the flavors to blend. Transfer the tuna tartare with avocado onto individual serving plates and serve as a fresh, light appetizer.

EGGS STUFFED WITH HAM

doses for 4 people

Ingredients:

6 eggs

100 g of raw ham

2 tablespoons mayonnaise

1 teaspoon Dijon mustard

1 teaspoon lemon juice

Salt and freshly ground black pepper

Chopped fresh parsley (optional)

Preparation:

Boil the eggs in salted water for about 10 minutes, then cool quickly under running cold water. Shell the eggs and cut them in half lengthwise. Remove the egg yolks and transfer them to a bowl. Finely chop the raw ham and add it to the egg yolks. Add the mayonnaise, Dijon mustard and lemon juice to the egg yolks and ham. Mix until you obtain a homogeneous consistency. Season with salt and freshly ground black pepper, adjusting to taste. Fill the egg halves with the egg yolk and ham mixture, using a teaspoon or piping bag. If desired, garnish with some chopped fresh parsley for a more attractive presentation. Arrange the stuffed eggs on a serving platter and serve as an appetizer or as part of a buffet.

MOZZARELLA AND SALAMI SKEWERS

Preparation time: approximately 15 minutes

Cooking time: approximately 1015 minutes

Ingredients:

doses for 4 people:

200 g of mozzarella

100 g of salami

1 red pepper

1 green pepper

1 red onion

Olive oil

Salt and Pepper To Taste

Rosemary sprigs (optional)

Preparation:

Cut the mozzarella and salami into similar sized cubes. Cut the peppers and onion into large pieces. Prepare the skewers by alternately threading the mozzarella, salami, peppers and onion cubes onto the wooden or metal skewers. Brush the skewers with a little olive oil and season with salt and pepper. If you wish, you can also add some sprigs of rosemary to further flavor the skewers. Preheat grill or nonstick skillet over medium-high heat. Cook the skewers for about 57 minutes on each side, turning them gently, until the mozzarella has melted and they have taken on a nice golden colour. Remove the skewers to the grill or pan and serve hot.

CRISPY CHICKEN LIVERS

Preparation time: approximately 10 minutes

Cooking time: approximately 1015 minutes

Ingredients:

doses for 4 people:

500 g of chicken livers

100 g of breadcrumbs

50 g of flour

2 eggs

Salt and Pepper To Taste

Vegetable oil for frying

Preparation:

Clean and dry the chicken livers, removing any skin or unwanted fatty parts.

In a bowl, break the eggs and beat them with salt and pepper. In a separate dish, mix together the breadcrumbs and flour. Dredge the livers first in the egg mixture and then in the breadcrumbs and flour mixture, making sure to cover them completely. Gently shake the livers to remove excess breadcrumbs. Heat plenty of vegetable oil in a pan over medium-high heat. Fry the livers in hot oil until golden and crisp, turning occasionally to ensure even cooking. It will take approximately 57 minutes. Once cooked, drain them on absorbent paper to remove excess oil. Serve the crispy chicken livers hot as an appetizer or accompaniment.

SMOKED CHICKEN SALAD WITH AVOCADO

Preparation time: approximately 15 minutes

Ingredients:

Doses for 4 people

2 smoked chicken breasts

2 ripe avocados

1 head of lettuce or mixed salad

1 tomato

1 cucumber

Lemon juice

Olive oil

Salt and Pepper To Taste

Fresh parsley (optional)

Preparation:

Cut the smoked chicken breast into cubes or strips. Peel and cut the avocados into cubes. Wash and cut the lettuce or mixed salad. Cut the tomato and cucumber into cubes. In a large bowl, combine the smoked chicken, avocados, lettuce, tomato and cucumber. Squeeze lemon juice over the salad and season with olive oil, salt and pepper to taste. Gently mix all ingredients until well combined. Add chopped fresh parsley on top of the salad, if desired. Serve the fresh and tasty Smoked Chicken Salad with Avocado.

BRUSCHETTA WITH TOMATO AND CRISPY BACON

Preparation time: approximately 18 minutes

Ingredients:

Doses for 4 people

4 slices of rustic bread

(like Tuscan bread or baguette)

2 ripe tomatoes

100 g of smoked bacon

2 cloves of garlic

Olive oil

Salt and Pepper To Taste

Fresh basil leaves (optional)

Preparation:

Heat a non-stick pan over medium heat and cook the bacon until crispy. Drain on absorbent paper to remove excess fat. Toast the slices of rustic bread lightly on both sides, until they become crispy. Peel the garlic cloves and rub lightly on the surface of the bread slices. Cut the tomatoes into cubes and place them in a bowl. Add olive oil, salt, pepper and chopped fresh basil to the tomatoes. Mix well. Place crispy bacon on bruschetta and then top with a generous portion of seasoned tomatoes. Repeat the process for the other slices of bread. Serve bruschetta with tomato and crispy bacon as an appetizer or snack.

FRESH NATURAL OYSTERS

Preparation time: approximately 10 minutes

Ingredients:

doses for 4 people:

16 fresh oysters

Preparation:

Choose good quality fresh oysters. Using an oyster knife or a sharp knife, gently open the oysters by removing the top lid. Remove any remaining shell from inside the oyster. Arrange the oysters on a serving platter with ice or on a bed of coarse salt to keep them fresh. Serve the oysters with lemon slices and mignonette sauce (a sauce made from wine vinegar, shallots and black pepper) or with a cocktail sauce, if you prefer.

SMOKED SALMON WITH CHEESE CREAM

45

Preparation time: approximately 15 minutes

Cooking time: none

Ingredients:

doses for 4 people:

200 g of smoked salmon

200 g of cream cheese

(e.g. Philadelphia)

Lemon juice

Fresh aromatic herbs

(such as dill or parsley)

Salt and Pepper To Taste

Preparation:

Cut the smoked salmon into thin slices. In a bowl, mix the cream cheese with lemon juice, chopped herbs, salt and pepper to taste. Make sure you get a smooth cream. Spread the cream cheese on the smoked salmon slices. Roll the salmon slices with the cream cheese and cut them into small rolls. Arrange the smoked salmon rolls with cream cheese on a serving plate. Decorate with additional fresh herbs. Serve as an appetizer.

MEAT PALLETS WITH BARBECUE SAUCE

Preparation time: approximately 20 minutes

Cooking time: approximately 25 minutes

ingredients

Doses for 4 people:

500g minced beef

1 egg

1/2 cup breadcrumbs

1/4 cup finely chopped onion

2 cloves of garlic finely chopped

2 tablespoons chopped fresh parsley

1/4 cup barbecue sauce

(plus extra for seasoning)

Salt and Pepper To Taste

Preparation

In a large bowl, combine the ground beef, egg, breadcrumbs, chopped onion, minced garlic, parsley, barbecue sauce, salt and pepper. Mix well until you obtain a uniform mixture. Prepare meatballs of the desired size, forming balls with your hands. R Heat a non-stick pan over medium-high heat and add a drizzle of oil. Place the meatballs in the pan and cook them for about 57 minutes on each side, until they are golden brown and cooked through. Once cooked, transfer the patties to a serving platter and top with additional barbecue sauce, if desired. Serve meatballs with barbecue sauce as an appetizer.

ASPARAGUS WRAPPED IN HAM

Preparation time: approximately 15 minutes

Cooking time: approximately 12 minutes

Ingredients:

Doses for 4 people:

16 fresh asparagus

8 slices of raw ham

Olive oil

Salt and Pepper To Taste

Preparation

Preheat the oven to 200°C. Take a bunch of asparagus and cut away the woody parts at the base of the stems. Wrap each asparagus with half a slice of raw ham, starting from the base to the tip. Arrange the asparagus wrapped in ham on a baking tray and season with a drizzle of olive oil, salt and pepper. Place the pan in the preheated oven and cook the asparagus for about 1012 minutes, until the ham is crispy and the asparagus is tender. Once cooked, transfer the ham-wrapped asparagus to a serving platter and serve hot. Ham-wrapped asparagus is delicious as an appetizer or side dish. You can accompany this preparation with a sauce based on mayonnaise, mustard or melted butter, if you want to further enrich the flavour.

CAPRESE SKEWERS WITH TOMATOES AND MOZZARELLA

Preparation time: approximately 15 minutes

Ingredients:

doses for 4 people

200 g of buffalo mozzarella

200 g of cherry tomatoes

Fresh basil leaves

Olive oil

Salt and Pepper To Taste

Skewers or toothpicks

Preparation:

Cut the buffalo mozzarella into cubes or spheres. Wash and dry the cherry tomatoes. Take a skewer or toothpick and insert a cherry tomato, then a cube or ball of mozzarella and a basil leaf. Repeat the operation until the ingredients are used up. Arrange the Caprese skewers on a serving plate. Season the skewers with a drizzle of olive oil, salt and pepper. Serve Caprese Skewers as an appetizer.

STARTERS OF MIXED CURED MEATS (SALAMI, HAM, COPPA)

Preparation time: approximately 1015 minutes

Ingredients:

doses for 4 people

100 g of salami

100 g of raw ham

100 g of coppa or other cured meat of your choice

Mixed olives, Chilies in oil (optional)

Preparation:

Cut the salami, raw ham and coppa into thin slices. Arrange the slices of cured meats on a serving plate. Add mixed olives and, if desired, pickled chili peppers to accompany the cured meats. Serve the appetizer of mixed cured meats with fresh bread or breadsticks.

SALMON CARPACCIO WITH HORSERADISH CREAM

Preparation time: approximately 15/20 minutes

doses for 4 people

Ingredients:

200 g of thinly sliced smoked salmon

Lemon juice

Olive oil

Salt and Pepper To Taste

2 tablespoons horseradish cream

Chopped fresh parsley (for garnish)

Preparation:

Arrange the smoked salmon slices on a serving plate. Squeeze the lemon juice over the salmon and season it with a drizzle of olive oil, salt and pepper. In a bowl, mix the horseradish cream with a teaspoon of lemon juice. Pour the horseradish cream over the salmon carpaccio, distributing evenly. Garnish the dish with chopped fresh parsley. Serve the salmon carpaccio with horseradish cream as an appetizer or as a light second course.

**PRAWN SKEWERS
WRAPPED IN BACON**

Preparation time: approximately 15/20 minutes

Cooking time: approximately 10 minutes

doses for 4 people

Ingredients:

16 fresh prawns, peeled and gutted

8 slices of bacon

Lemon juice

Olive oil

Salt and Pepper To Taste

Skewers or toothpicks

Preparation:

Preheat the oven grill or barbecue. Wrap each shrimp with half a slice of bacon. Thread the bacon-wrapped shrimp onto skewers or toothpicks. Season the skewers with lemon juice, olive oil, salt and pepper. Cook the bacon-wrapped shrimp skewers under the oven broiler or on the barbecue grill for about 8/10 minutes, turning occasionally, until the bacon is crispy and the shrimp are cooked through. Once cooked, transfer the bacon-wrapped shrimp skewers to a serving platter and serve hot.

GOOSE LIVER PATÉ CANAPES

Preparation time: approximately 10/15 minutes

doses for 4 people

Ingredients:

150 g of goose liver pâté

Slices of bread (baguette or toast)

Salt and Pepper To Taste

Fruit jam to taste

(figs or currants optional)

Preparation:

Spread the goose liver pâté on the bread slices. If desired, spread a little butter on the bread slices before adding the pate. Season with salt and pepper to taste. You can serve the pâté canapés as they are or you can accompany with a spoonful of fruit jam to add a sweet note.

BREADED CHICKEN BITES

Preparation time: approximately 20/25 minutes

Cooking time: approximately 15/20 minutes

doses for 4 people

Ingredients:

500g chicken breast, cut into bite-sized pieces

Flour to taste

2 eggs, beaten

Breadcrumbs to taste

Salt and Pepper To Taste

Vegetable oil for frying

Preparation:

Prepare a small bowl with the flour, another with the beaten eggs and a third with the breadcrumbs. Season the chicken pieces with salt and pepper. Dip each morsel in the flour, then in the beaten egg and finally in the breadcrumbs, making sure to cover each piece well. Heat plenty of vegetable oil in a pan. Fry the chicken tenders over medium-high heat until golden brown and crispy, about 57 minutes per side. Once cooked, transfer the chicken pieces to absorbent paper to remove excess oil. Serve the breaded chicken pieces with sauces such as barbecue sauce or mayonnaise.

BOILED EGGS WITH CRISPY BACON

Preparation time: approximately 10 minutes

Cooking time: approximately 10/12 minutes

doses for 4 people

Ingredients:

4 eggs

8 slices of bacon

Salt and Pepper To Taste

Fresh herbs (such as

parsley or thyme, optional)

Preparation:

Bring a pot of water to a boil and carefully add the eggs. Cook the eggs for about 10/12 minutes to get hard boiled eggs. While the eggs are cooking, heat a nonstick skillet over medium-high heat and cook the bacon slices until crisp. You can cook bacon without adding oil, as the bacon fat will melt during cooking. Drain the bacon on absorbent paper to remove excess fat. Shell the hard-boiled eggs, cut in half lengthwise and season them with a pinch of salt and pepper. Wrap each hard-boiled egg half with a slice of crispy bacon. If you wish, you can garnish with fresh herbs such as parsley or thyme. Serve hard-boiled eggs with bacon as an appetizer.

ZUCCHINI ROLLS WITH HAM AND CHEESE

Preparation time: approximately 20 minutes

Cooking time: approximately 10/12 minutes

doses for 4 people

Ingredients:

2 medium courgettes

4 slices of raw ham

Fresh cheese to taste

Olive oil

Salt and Pepper To Taste

Preparation:

Preheat the oven to 200°C. Trim the ends of the courgettes and cut them into long, thin slices lengthwise.

Brush the courgette slices with a drizzle of olive oil and season with salt and pepper. Place a slice of raw ham on each courgette slice and add a little cheese on top of the ham. Roll up the courgette slices with the ham and cheese inside, forming rolls. Place the courgette rolls on a baking tray and cook them in the preheated oven for about 10/12 minutes, until the courgettes are soft and the ham is crispy. Once cooked, transfer the courgette rolls to a serving plate and serve hot as an appetizer or side dish.

COOKED HAM
WITH FRESH FIGS

Preparation time: approximately 15 minutes

Cooking time: none

doses for 4 people

Ingredients:

8 slices of cooked ham

4 fresh figs, cut in half

Cheese to taste (like cheese

goat or gorgonzola)

Honey to taste

Arugula (optional)

Preparation:

Arrange the slices of cooked ham on a serving plate. Place a fig half on each slice of ham. Add a little cheese to the top of each fig. You can also add a drizzle of honey over the figs and cheese for a touch of sweetness. If you wish, you can add a bed of rocket on the serving plate and place the slices of cooked ham with figs on top. Serve the cooked ham with fresh figs as an appetizer or as part of a mixed salad.

VEAL CHOPS STUFFED WITH CHEESE AND OLIVES

Preparation time: approximately 15/20 minutes

Cooking time: approximately 20/25 minutes

doses for 4 people

Ingredients:

4 thin veal chops

Stretched curd cheese cut into thin slices

Pitted green olives, chopped

Bread crumbs

Eggs, beaten, Flour

Salt and Pepper To Taste

Olive oil for cooking

Preparation:

Prepare thin veal chops and season them with salt and pepper on both sides. Spread a slice of cheese and some chopped olives over the veal chops. Roll the stuffed chops on themselves and secure them with a toothpick to keep them closed. Prepare three dishes: one with the flour, one with the beaten eggs and one with the breadcrumbs. Dip the stuffed chops in the flour, then in the beaten egg and finally in the breadcrumbs, making sure to coat each piece well. Heat some olive oil in a nonstick skillet over medium-high heat. Add the stuffed chops to the pan and cook for about 1012 minutes per side, until golden brown and cooked through. Once cooked, transfer the stuffed chops to a serving plate and serve hot.

CHICKEN SALAD WITH WALNUTS AND MUSTARD SAUCE

Preparation time: 15 minutes

Cooking time: 20 minutes

Ingredients

(for 4 people):

2 skinless chicken breasts

4 cups mixed lettuce

1 cup chopped walnuts

1/2 cup diced celery

1/2 cup raisins

1/4 cup mayonnaise

2 tablespoons of mustard

1 tablespoon lemon juice

Salt and Pepper To Taste

Preparation:

Preheat the oven to 180°C. Brush the chicken breasts with a little olive oil and season with salt and pepper. Bake the chicken breasts in the preheated oven for 20 minutes, or until cooked through. Once cooked, let them cool for a few minutes. Meanwhile, prepare the mustard sauce. In a bowl, mix the mayonnaise, mustard, lemon juice, salt and pepper. Dice the cooked chicken. In a large bowl, combine the lettuce, chopped walnuts, diced celery, raisins and diced chicken. Pour the mustard sauce over the mixture and mix well to evenly distribute the sauce. Taste the salad and add salt and pepper if necessary. Serve the chicken salad with walnuts and mustard dressing as a light appetizer.

GRILLED SAUSAGES
WITH MUSTARD

Preparation time: 5 minutes

Cooking time: 10/15 minutes

Ingredients

(for 4 people):

8 sausages (you can choose the type

of sausage you prefer)

4 tablespoons of mustard

2 tablespoons honey

1 tablespoon olive oil

Salt and Pepper To Taste

Preparation:

Preheat the grill or barbecue to medium-high. In a bowl, mix the mustard, honey, olive oil, salt and pepper. Brush the sausages with the mustard mixture and place on the preheated grill. Cook the sausages for 57 minutes per side, or until cooked through and have nice grilled streaks. While cooking, brush the sausages with some of the remaining mustard mixture to intensify the flavor. Once cooked, remove the sausages to the grill and let them rest for a few minutes. Serve the grilled sausages with mustard accompanied by side dishes of your choice, such as bread, fries or grilled vegetables.

BACON AND CHEESE OMELETTE

Preparation time: 10 minutes

Cooking time: 15 minutes

Ingredients

(for 2 people):

4 slices of smoked bacon

4 eggs

1/4 cup milk

100 g of grated cheese

Salt and Pepper To Taste

2 tablespoons of olive oil

Preparation:

In a non-stick pan, cook the smoked bacon until crispy. Once cooked, drain it on paper absorbent to eliminate excess fat and cut it into small pieces. In a bowl, beat the eggs with the milk. Add the grated cheese, chopped bacon, salt and pepper. Mix all the ingredients well. Heat the olive oil in the same pan you cooked the bacon in. Pour the egg mixture into the pan and spread evenly. Cook the omelette over medium-low heat for 15 minutes, or until it is well set around the edges and slightly soft in the centre. When the omelette is ready, gently shake it in the pan to make sure it doesn't stick. Using a lid or a plate, flip the omelette to cook the other side as well. Cook it for another 23 minutes. Transfer the omelette to a serving plate and cut it into wedges. Serve hot.

BEEF TARTARE WITH EGG YOLK

Preparation time: 15 minutes

Ingredients

(for 2 people):

300g minced beef

1 fresh egg yolk

1 tablespoon Dijon mustard

1 teaspoon Worcestershire sauce

1 teaspoon soy sauce

1/2 red onion, finely chopped

Chopped fresh parsley to taste

Salt and Pepper To Taste

Preparation:

In a bowl, combine the ground beef, Dijon mustard, Worcestershire sauce, soy sauce, chopped red onion, fresh parsley, salt and pepper. Make sure you mix all the ingredients well. Divide the seasoned meat into two equal portions and shape them into two flat discs on the surface of the serving plates. With the back of a spoon, create a small indentation in the center of each disc of meat. Place a fresh egg yolk in the center of each well. Garnish the tartare with a pinch of chopped fresh parsley and some additional salt and pepper to taste. Serve the beef tartare with egg yolk with toast or croutons, so that guests can spread the seasoned meat on top.

CURRY CHICKEN SKEWERS

Preparation time: 15 minutes

Cooking time: 10/15 minutes

Ingredients

(for 4 people):

2 chicken breasts, cut into cubes

2 tablespoons of olive oil

2 tablespoons curry powder

Juice of 1 lemon

Salt and Pepper To Taste

8 x Skewer Sticks

Preparation:

In a bowl, mix the olive oil, curry powder, lemon juice, salt and pepper. Add the chicken cubes to the marinade and toss well to coat evenly. Leave to marinate for at least 30 minutes, but if you have more time you can leave the chicken to marinate for several hours for a more intense flavor. Preheat your grill or barbecue to medium-high. Thread the marinated chicken cubes onto the skewers, distributing evenly. Grill the chicken skewers for 10/15 minutes, turning occasionally, until well cooked and lightly browned. Once cooked, serve the hot chicken curry skewers as an appetizer with a sauce of your choice.

CROSTINI WITH MEAT PATÉ

Preparation time: 10 minutes

Cooking time: 15/20 minutes

Ingredients

(for about 8 croutons):

200 g of minced beef

1 small onion, finely chopped

1 clove garlic, finely chopped

2 tablespoons of olive oil

2 tablespoons of tomato paste

1 teaspoon sweet paprika

Salt and Pepper To Taste

Toast or crostini for serving

Preparation:

In a skillet, heat the olive oil over medium heat. Add the chopped onion and garlic and cook for a few minutes until soft and translucent. Add the ground beef to the pan and cook until fully cooked and browned. Be sure to break up any lumps of meat while cooking. Add tomato paste and sweet paprika to the minced meat. Mix well to incorporate the ingredients. Cook the meat pâté over medium-low heat for another 5 minutes, stirring occasionally. Make sure all the ingredients are well combined and the pâté is well seasoned. Add salt and pepper to your taste. Toast bread or make croutons. Spread the meat pâté generously on the croutons or toast. Serve the crostini with meat pâté as an appetizer or appetizer.

PORK PINCHOS WITH CHILI SAUCE

Preparation time: 15 minutes

Cooking time: 10/15 minutes

Ingredients

(for 4 people):

500g diced pork

1 tablespoon olive oil

1 tablespoon smoked paprika

1 teaspoon garlic powder

Salt and pepper to taste, 8 skewer sticks

For the chili sauce:

2 hot red chillies

2 tablespoons of olive oil

Juice of 1 lemon, Salt to taste

Preparation:

Preheat your grill or barbecue to medium-high. In a bowl, toss the pork cubes with olive oil, smoked paprika, garlic powder, salt and pepper. Mix well to coat the meat evenly. Thread seasoned pork cubes onto skewers, distributing evenly. Grill the pork pinchos for 10/15 minutes, turning them occasionally, until they are well cooked and lightly browned. Meanwhile, prepare the chili sauce. Finely chop the hot red chillies and place them in a bowl. Add the olive oil, lemon juice and salt. Mix well to combine the ingredients. Once cooked, serve the pork pinchos hot with the chili sauce as a condiment or dipping sauce.

POACHED EGGS WITH CRISPY BACON

Preparation time: 10 minutes

Cooking time: 10 minutes

Ingredients

(for 2 people):

4 eggs

4 slices of bacon

1 tablespoon white wine vinegar

Salt and Pepper To Taste

Chopped fresh parsley

for garnish (optional)

Preparation:

In a nonstick skillet, cook the bacon over medium-high heat until crisp.

Drain on absorbent paper to remove excess fat. Fill a pot with water and bring it to a boil. Add the white wine vinegar and a pinch of salt. Gently crack an egg into a separate cup. Create a vortex in the boiling water with a spoon and pour the egg into the center of the vortex. Repeat the process with the other eggs, one at a time. Poach the eggs for about 34 minutes, until the yolks are still soft but the eggs are set. Using a slotted spoon, gently remove the eggs from the boiling water and place them on absorbent paper to remove excess water. Arrange the crispy bacon slices on a serving plate. Place the poached eggs on top. Season the eggs with salt and pepper to taste. If desired, garnish with some chopped fresh parsley. Serve poached eggs with crispy bacon.

TURKEY BITES WITH YOGURT AND GARLIC SAUCE

Preparation time: 15 minutes

Cooking time: 10/15 minutes

Ingredients

(for 4 people):

500 g of turkey nuggets

2 tablespoons olive oil, Juice of 1 lemon

2 cloves garlic, finely chopped

1 teaspoon dried oregano

Salt and Pepper To Taste

For the yogurt and garlic sauce:

200g Greek yogurt, 1 clove of garlic, chopped

Chopped fresh parsley to taste

Salt and pepper to taste Juice of 1/2 lemon

Preparation:

In a bowl, mix the olive oil, lemon juice, minced garlic, dried oregano, salt and pepper. Add the turkey tenders to the marinade and toss well to coat them evenly. Leave to marinate for at least 30 minutes, but if you have more time you can leave the turkey to marinate for several hours for a more intense flavor. Pre Heat a skillet or grill over medium-high heat. Cook the turkey pieces for 10/15 minutes, turning them occasionally, until they are well cooked and golden. Meanwhile, prepare the yogurt and garlic sauce. In a bowl, mix Greek yogurt, minced garlic, lemon juice, chopped fresh parsley, salt and pepper. Stir well to combine the ingredients. Once the turkey pieces are cooked, serve hot accompanied by the yogurt and garlic sauce as a condiment.

TUNA SALAD WITH OLIVES AND TOMATOES

Preparation time: 10 minutes

Ingredients

(for 4 people):

2 cans canned tuna, drained

200g cherry tomatoes, cut in half

100 g black olives, pitted

1 red onion, thinly sliced

Chopped fresh parsley to taste

Juice of 1 lemon

3 tablespoons of olive oil

Salt and Pepper To Taste

Preparation:

In a bowl, crumble the canned tuna with a fork. Add the cherry tomatoes cut in half, the pitted black olives and the sliced red onion. Gently mix the ingredients. Season the tuna salad with chopped fresh parsley, lemon juice, olive oil, salt and pepper. Stir well to combine the ingredients and make sure the salad is well seasoned. Serve the tuna salad with olives and cherry tomatoes.

SAUSAGE MEATBALLS WITH MARINARA SAUCE

Preparation time: 15 minutes

Cooking time: 20/25 minutes

Ingredients

(for 4 people):

500 g of fresh sausage, without skin

1 egg, 100 g of breadcrumbs

100 g grated parmesan cheese

2 tablespoons chopped fresh parsley

1/2 teaspoon garlic powder

Salt and Pepper To Taste

Olive oil for cooking

For the marinara sauce:

2 cups tomato puree

1 clove garlic, finely chopped

1/2 teaspoon dried oregano

Salt and Pepper To Taste

Preparation:

In a bowl, break the fresh sausage and crumble it. Add the egg, breadcrumbs, grated cheese, chopped parsley, garlic powder, salt and pepper. Mix the ingredients well until you obtain a homogeneous mixture. Shape the sausage mixture into round patties and arrange on a plate. Pre Heat a pan with a little olive oil over medium-high heat. Add the sausage patties to the pan and cook them for about 10/12 minutes, turning them occasionally, until they are well cooked and golden on all sides. Meanwhile, prepare the marinara sauce. In a saucepan, heat the tomato puree together with the chopped garlic, oregano, salt and pepper. Cook over medium heat for 57 minutes, until the sauce is heated through and the flavors blend. Transfer the sausage meatballs to the pan with the marinara sauce and let them cook for another 5/10 minutes over medium-low heat, so that they flavor and blend with the sauce. Serve sausage patties with marinara sauce as an appetizer.

AUBERGINES ROLLS WITH HAM AND CHEESE

Preparation time: 15 minutes

Cooking time: 20/25 minutes

Ingredients

(for 4 people):

2 large aubergines

8 slices of raw ham

200 g of sliced cheese

2 cups marinara sauce

Olive oil for cooking

Salt and Pepper To Taste

Preparation:

Cut the aubergines into thin slices, lengthwise, about half a centimeter thick.

Heat a grill or nonstick skillet over medium-high heat. Brush the aubergine slices with a little olive oil and grill for about 23 minutes per side, until tender and lightly browned. Add salt and pepper during cooking. Take a slice of grilled aubergine and place it on a cutting board. Arrange a slice of raw ham and a slice of cheese on top. Roll the aubergine around the ham and cheese to form a roll. Repeat the process with the other eggplant slices. Place the aubergine rolls on a baking tray lightly greased with olive oil. Pour the marinara sauce over the surface of the eggplant rolls. Bake the pan in the preheated oven at 180°C and cook the aubergine rolls for about 15/20 minutes, until the cheese melts and the sauce heats up. Serve the eggplant rolls with ham and cheese as an appetizer.

SALMON MARINATED WITH AROMATIC HERBS

Preparation time: 10 minutes

(marinating: 30/60 minutes)

Ingredients

(for 4 people):

500 g of salmon fillet

fresh, skinless

Juice of 2 lemons

Grated zest of 1 lemon

2 tablespoons fresh herbs

chopped (for example parsley,

basil, chives)

2 tablespoons of olive oil

Salt and Pepper To Taste

Preparation:

Cut the salmon fillet into thin slices and arrange them on a serving plate. In a bowl, combine the lemon juice, grated lemon zest, chopped herbs, olive oil, salt and pepper. Mix the ingredients well to obtain a marinade. Pour the marinade over the salmon slices, making sure they are well covered on all sides. Cover the dish with cling film and leave to marinate in the refrigerator for at least 30/60 minutes, so that the salmon absorbs the flavors of the herbs and lemon. Once marinated, you can serve the herb-marinated salmon as an appetizer. You can garnish with some chopped fresh herbs and thin slices of lemon.

STARTER BRESAOLA WITH ARUGULA AND GRANA FLAKES

Preparation time: 10 minutes

Ingredients

(for 4 people):

200 g of thinly sliced bresaola

2 handfuls of fresh Arugula

100 g of parmesan flakes

Juice of 1 lemon

Extra virgin olive oil to taste

Salt and Pepper To Taste

Preparation:

Take individual plates or a serving plate and arrange the bresaola slices decoratively. Distribute the arugula evenly over the bresaola slices. Add the parmesan flakes to the Arugula. Squeeze lemon juice over the appetizer and drizzle with extra virgin olive oil. Add salt and pepper to your taste. Serve the bresaola appetizer with rocket and parmesan flakes as a first course or as a light appetizer.

OVEN GRATINATED OYSTERS

Preparation time: 15 minutes

Cooking time: 10/12 minutes

Ingredients

(for 4 people):

12 fresh oysters

2 tablespoons melted butter

1 clove garlic, finely chopped

1/4 cup breadcrumbs

100 g grated parmesan cheese

Chopped fresh parsley to taste

Salt and Pepper To Taste

Lemon slices for garnish

Preparation:

Preheat the oven to 220°C. Shuck the oysters from their shells, taking care to collect and preserve any juice they may release. In a bowl, mix the melted butter, minced garlic, breadcrumbs, grated cheese, chopped parsley, salt and pepper. Mix well to form a compact paste. Place the oysters on the rack of a heatproof oven or on a lightly greased baking tray. Cover each oyster with a generous teaspoon of the breadcrumb and cheese mixture. Bake the gratin oysters in the oven for 10/12 minutes, until the surface becomes golden and crunchy. Remove from the oven and serve the gratin oysters hot, garnished with lemon slices.

STUFFED POTATOES WITH BACON AND CHEESE

Preparation time: 15 minutes

Cooking time: 1 hour

Ingredients

(for 4 people):

4 large potatoes

100g bacon, cut into cubes

1/2 cup grated cheese

1/4 cup heavy cream

2 tablespoons melted butter

Chopped parsley to taste, Salt and pepper to taste

Preparation:

Preheat the oven to 200°C. Wash the potatoes well and dry them. Make deep cuts lengthwise across the top of each potato. Wrap the potatoes in foil and place them on a baking sheet. Cook in the oven for about 45/50 minutes, until the potatoes are tender. Meanwhile, in a skillet, cook the bacon over medium heat until crisp. Drain on absorbent paper to remove excess oil. Remove the potatoes from the oven and let them cool slightly. Cut off the tops of the potatoes and gently empty the pulp into a bowl. Mash the potato pulp with a fork and add the grated cheese, cooking cream, crispy bacon, melted butter, chopped parsley, salt and pepper. Mix all the ingredients well until you obtain a homogeneous mixture. Fill the potatoes with the bacon and cheese mixture, pressing well. Place the stuffed potatoes back into the baking tray and cook in the oven for another 10/15 minutes, until the surface becomes golden. Remove from the oven and serve the potatoes stuffed with bacon and cheese hot.

CHICKEN SALAD WITH CUCUMBERS AND AVOCADO

Preparation time: 15 minutes

Ingredients

(for 4 people):

2 cooked chicken breasts, cut into cubes

1 cucumber, cut into thin slices

1 ripe avocado, cut into cubes

1 cup cherry tomatoes, cut in half

1/4 red onion, thinly sliced

Juice of 1 lemon

2 tablespoons of olive oil

Chopped fresh parsley to taste

Salt and Pepper To Taste

Preparation:

In a large bowl, combine the diced chicken, sliced cucumbers, diced avocado, halved cherry tomatoes and sliced red onion. In a small bowl, mix the lemon juice, olive oil, chopped fresh parsley, salt and pepper. Pour this vinaigrette over the chicken and vegetable mixture and stir gently to combine the ingredients well. Let the chicken salad with cucumber and avocado rest in the refrigerator for at least 30 minutes before serving, so that the flavors blend well. Serve the light chicken salad. You can garnish with some chopped fresh parsley.

HAM AND CHEESE FLADS

Preparation time: 10 minutes

Cooking time: 20/25 minutes

Ingredients

(for 4 people):

8 slices of raw ham

200 g of cheese (mozzarella,

provolone or cheddar), cut into cubes

4 eggs, 1/2 cup milk

Salt and Pepper To Taste

olive oil to grease the molds

Preparation:

Preheat the oven to 180°C. Take some soufflé molds or individual baking cups and lightly grease the inside surface with olive oil.

Line each mold with 2 slices of ham, so that the slices overlap and completely cover the internal surface of the mold. Place a few cubes of cheese inside each ham-lined mold. In a bowl, beat the eggs with the milk, salt and pepper. Gently pour this mixture into the molds, spreading evenly over the cheese cubes. Place the molds on a baking tray and bake in the preheated oven for 20/25 minutes, or until the ham and cheese flans are puffy and golden on the surface. Remove the flans from the oven and let them cool slightly before removing them from the molds. Serve the ham and cheese flans, accompanying them with a fresh green salad or grilled vegetables.

RECIPES
FIRST DISHES

SPAGHETTI CARBONARA

Preparation time: 10 minutes

Cooking time: 10/12 minutes

Ingredients

(for 4 people):

400 g of spaghetti

200 g of bacon or bacon

smoked, cut into cubes

4 egg yolks

100 g of pecorino cheese

grated romano

Salt to taste

Freshly ground black pepper to taste

Preparation:

Start by bringing a pot of salted water to a boil. Cook the spaghetti according to package instructions, until al dente. Meanwhile, in a large pan, brown the bacon or bacon cubes over medium-high heat until golden and crisp. Remove the pan from the heat. In a bowl, beat the egg yolks with the grated pecorino romano cheese. Add a generous grind of black pepper and mix well. Drain the spaghetti al dente, keeping a little of the cooking water. Add the spaghetti to the pan with the bacon or bacon and mix well to flavor them with the meat fat.

Remove the pan from the heat and add the egg and cheese mixture, stirring vigorously to combine the ingredients. Add a little spaghetti cooking water if the pasta is too dry. Make sure the egg and cheese sauce has thickened and coats the spaghetti well. Serve the spaghetti carbonara hot, garnished with a sprinkling of grated pecorino romano cheese and freshly ground black pepper.

LASAGNA BOLOGNESE

Preparation time: 30 minutes

Cooking time: 45 minutes

Ingredients

(for 4 people):

12 sheets of lasagna pasta

500 g of minced meat

(mixed beef and pork)

1 onion, finely chopped

2 cloves garlic, finely chopped

400 g of tomato pulp

2 tablespoons of tomato paste

1/2 cup red wine

1 cup of milk

1/2 cup beef broth

50 g of butter,

50 g of flour

200 g of grated parmesan cheese

Salt and Pepper To Taste

Nutmeg to taste

Preparation:

Start by preparing the Bolognese ragù. In a large skillet, sauté the onion and garlic with a little olive oil until translucent. Add the ground beef to the pan and cook until well browned and free of liquid. Add the tomato pulp, tomato paste and red wine. Mix well and leave to cook over medium-low heat for about 15/20 minutes, until the ragù has thickened. Add the milk and meat broth to the ragù. Mix well and let cook for another 10 minutes. Add salt, pepper and nutmeg to taste. Keep aside

Bolognese ragù. In a separate pan, prepare the béchamel sauce. Melt the butter over medium heat, then add the flour and stir vigorously to form a roux. Gradually add the milk, stirring constantly to avoid lumps. Continue stirring until the béchamel thickens. Add about 1/4 cup shredded cheese and stir until completely melted. Keep the béchamel sauce aside. Preheat the oven to 180°C. In a rectangular baking pan, start assembling the lasagna. Start with a layer of Bolognese sauce, followed by a sheet of lasagna pasta, then a layer of bechamel. Continue alternating layers until you run out of ingredients, finishing with a layer of béchamel sauce and a generous sprinkling of grated cheese on top. Cover the pan with foil and bake for about 30 minutes. Remove the foil and cook for another 10/15 minutes, until the surface is golden and crispy. Remove from the oven and let the lasagna rest for a few minutes before serving.

GNOCCHI WITH MEAT SAUCE

Preparation time: 10 minutes

Cooking time: 30 minutes

Ingredients

(for 4 people):

500 g of gnocchi

400 g of minced meat

(mixed beef and pork)

1 onion, finely chopped

2 cloves garlic, finely chopped

400 g of tomato pulp

2 tablespoons of tomato paste

1/2 cup red wine

1/2 cup beef broth

2 tablespoons of olive oil

Salt and Pepper To Taste

Grated cheese for garnish

Chopped fresh parsley for garnish (optional)

Preparation:

Start by preparing the meat sauce. In a skillet, heat the olive oil over medium heat and add the onion and garlic. Sauté until translucent. Add the ground beef to the pan and cook until well browned and free of liquid. Add the tomato pulp, tomato paste and red wine.

Mix well and leave to cook over medium-low heat for about 15/20 minutes, until the ragù has thickened. Add the meat broth to the ragù and let it cook for another 5 minutes. Add salt and pepper to taste. Meanwhile, bring a pot of salted water to a boil. Cook the gnocchi according to package instructions, until al dente. Drain the gnocchi and add them to the meat sauce. Mix gently to make them flavor with the ragù. Serve the gnocchi with ragù hot, garnished with grated cheese and chopped fresh parsley if desired.

LENTIL SOUP WITH SAUSAGE

Preparation time: 10 minutes

Cooking time: 40/50 minutes

Ingredients

(for 46 people):

250 g of dried lentils

2 sausages, peeled and crumbled

1 onion, finely chopped

2 carrots, diced

2 stalks celery, diced

2 cloves garlic, finely chopped

1 bay leaf

1 liter of vegetable broth or meat broth

2 tablespoons of olive oil

Salt and Pepper To Taste

Chopped fresh parsley for garnish

Preparation:

Start by rinsing the lentils under running water and stirring them. In a large pot, heat the olive oil over medium heat and add the onion, carrots, celery and garlic. Sauté until the vegetables begin to soften. Add the crumbled sausage to the pot and cook until well browned. Add the lentils, bay leaf and vegetable broth or beef broth. Bring to the boil, then reduce the heat to medium-low, cover the pan and cook for about 30/40 minutes, until the lentils are soft and tender. Add salt and pepper to taste. Remove the bay leaf from the soup and serve hot, garnished with chopped fresh parsley.

RISOTTO MILANESE WITH OSSOBUCO

Preparation time: 15 minutes

Cooking time: 1 hour and 30 minutes

Ingredients

(for 4 people):

320 g of Carnaroli or Arborio rice

4 veal ossobucco

1 onion, finely chopped

2 cloves garlic, finely chopped

1/2 cup dry white wine

1.5 l of meat broth

Saffron pistils (one sachet)

50 g of butter, Salt and pepper to taste

50 g grated parmesan cheese

Preparation:

Start by preparing the osso buco. In a large pot, heat some olive oil and add the onion and garlic. Sauté until translucent. Add the shanks to the pan and brown them on both sides until golden brown. Add the white wine and let it evaporate for a few minutes. Add the beef broth to the pot, cover it with a lid and let it cook over low heat for about 1 hour and 15 minutes, until the meat is tender and comes away easily from the bones. Meanwhile, prepare the risotto. In a separate saucepan, melt the butter over medium heat. Add the rice and toast it for a few minutes, stirring constantly. Add a ladle of hot broth to the rice and stir until absorbed.

Continue adding the broth, a little at a time, stirring constantly, until the rice is al dente and creamy. This should take around 15/20 minutes. Add the saffron to the risotto and mix well to distribute it evenly. Remove the osso buco from the pot, remove the bone and cut the meat into slices or stracciatella. Add the osso buco meat to the risotto and mix gently. Add the grated cheese to the risotto and stir until it melts completely. Add salt and pepper to taste. Serve the Milanese risotto with hot osso buco, garnished with a sprinkling of grated cheese.

PENNE ALL'ARRABBIATA WITH BACON

Preparation time: 10 minutes

Cooking time: 20 minutes

Ingredients

(for 4 people):

320 g of penne

200 g of smoked bacon,

cut into cubes

1 onion, finely chopped

2 cloves garlic, finely chopped

400 g of peeled tomatoes

1/2 cup dry white wine

Fresh chili pepper, chopped

Olive oil to taste Salt to taste

Chopped fresh parsley for garnish

Preparation:

Start by making the arrabiata sauce. In a large pan, heat some olive oil and add the bacon. Cook it until golden and crispy. Add the onion and garlic to the pan and sauté until translucent. Add the peeled tomatoes to the pan, mashing them lightly with a fork. Add white wine and chilli to taste. Let it cook over medium-low heat for about 15/20 minutes, until the sauce has thickened. Meanwhile, bring a pot of salted water to the boil and cook the penne according to the package instructions, until al dente. Drain the penne and add them to the pan with the arrabiata sauce. Mix well to flavor them with the sauce. Serve the penne all'Arrabbiata hot, garnished with fresh chopped parsley.

CANNELLONI STUFFED WITH MEAT

Preparation time: 20 minutes

Cooking time: 30/35 minutes

Ingredients

(for 4 people):

12 dried cannelloni

300g minced beef

1 onion, finely chopped

2 cloves garlic, finely chopped

400 g of tomato pulp

2 tablespoons of tomato paste

1/2 cup red wine

1 cup of bechamel

1/2 cup grated Parmesan cheese

2 tablespoons of olive oil

Salt and Pepper To Taste

Chopped fresh parsley for garnish

Preparation:

Start by preparing the meat filling. In a skillet, heat the olive oil over medium heat and add the onion and garlic. Sauté until translucent. Add the ground beef to the pan and cook until well browned and free of liquid. Add the tomato pulp, tomato paste and red wine. Mix well and leave to cook over medium-low heat for about 15/20 minutes, until the sauce has thickened. Add salt and pepper to taste. In the meantime, bring a pan of salted water to the boil and cook the cannelloni following the instructions on the package, until they are al dente. Drain the cannelloni and let them cool slightly. Fill them with the prepared meat filling. Preheat the oven to 180°C. Prepare a rectangular baking pan and spread a layer of béchamel sauce on the bottom. Place the stuffed cannelloni on the baking tray, arranging them in a single layer. Pour the remaining béchamel sauce over the cannelloni and sprinkle the grated cheese on top. Bake for about 15/20 minutes, until the cheese is golden and crunchy. Remove from the oven and let the cannelloni rest for a few minutes before serving. Sprinkle with fresh chopped parsley before serving.

TAGLIATELLE WITH BOAR SAUCE

Preparation time: 15 minutes

Cooking time: 1 hour and 30 minutes

Ingredients

(for 4 people):

320 g of tagliatelle

500 g of chopped wild boar meat

1 onion, finely chopped

2 cloves garlic, finely chopped

400 g of tomato pulp

2 tablespoons of tomato paste

1/2 cup red wine

2 tablespoons of olive oil

Salt and Pepper To Taste

Chopped fresh parsley for garnish

Preparation:

Start by preparing the wild boar ragù. In a large pot, heat the olive oil over medium heat and add the onion and garlic. Sauté until translucent. Add the chopped wild boar meat to the pot and cook until well browned and free of liquid. Add the tomato pulp, tomato paste and red wine. Mix well and leave to cook over medium-low heat for about 1 hour and 30 minutes, until the ragù has thickened. Add salt and pepper to taste. Meanwhile, bring a pot of salted water to the boil and cook the tagliatelle according to the package instructions, until al dente. Drain the tagliatelle and season them with the prepared wild boar ragù. Serve the tagliatelle with wild boar ragù hot, garnished with fresh chopped parsley.

BEAN SOUP WITH HAM

Preparation time: 10 minutes

Cooking time: 1 hour and 30 minutes

Ingredients

(for 4 people):

250 g of dried cannellini beans

100 g of raw ham, cut into cubes

1 onion, finely chopped

2 cloves garlic, finely chopped

2 carrots, cut into cubes

2 stalks celery, cut into cubes

1 bay leaf

1 liter vegetable broth or chicken broth

2 tablespoons olive oil, Salt and pepper to taste

Chopped fresh parsley for garnish

Preparation:

Start by preparing the beans. Place the dried beans in a bowl and cover them with plenty of cold water. Let them soak for at least 8 hours or overnight. Drain and rinse them well under running water. In a large pot, heat the olive oil over medium heat and add the onion and garlic. Sauté until translucent. Add the ham, carrots and celery to the pot and continue to cook for a few minutes. Add the soaked beans, bay leaf, and vegetable broth or chicken broth to the pot. Bring to the boil, then reduce the heat to medium-low, cover the pot and simmer for about 1 hour 30 minutes, until the beans are soft and the soup has thickened. Add salt and pepper to taste. Remove the bay leaf from the soup and serve hot, garnished with chopped fresh parsley.

MEAT RAVIOLI WITH BUTTER AND SAGE

Preparation time: 5 minutes

Cooking time: 57 minutes

Ingredients

(for 4 people):

250 g of fresh meat ravioli

50 g of butter

Fresh sage leaves

Salt to taste

Grated parmesan cheese

Preparation:

Bring a pot of salted water to the boil and cook the ravioli according to the package instructions, until al dente. Meanwhile, melt the butter in a pan over medium-low heat. Add the sage leaves to the pan and fry them for a few minutes, until they become crispy. Drain the ravioli and transfer them to the pan with the butter and sage. Toss gently to coat the ravioli with the butter and sage. Serve the meat ravioli with hot butter and sage, sprinkling with grated cheese.

BAKED MACARONI WITH MEATBALLS

Preparation time: 10 minutes

Cooking time: 30/35 minutes

Ingredients

(for 4 people):

350 g of macaroni

400 g of meatballs

500 ml of tomato sauce

200 g mozzarella, cut into cubes

50 g of grated cheese

2 tablespoons of olive oil

Salt and Pepper To Taste

Chopped fresh parsley for garnish

Preparation:

Start by making the meatballs. If you are using frozen meatballs, follow the instructions on the package for cooking them. Bring a pot of salted water to the boil and cook the macaroni according to the package instructions, until al dente. Meanwhile, in a pan, heat the olive oil over medium heat and add the tomato sauce. Let it warm up for a few minutes. Add the meatballs to the pan with the tomato sauce and let them cook for about 10/15 minutes, until they are cooked and the sauce has thickened slightly. Preheat the oven to 180°C. Drain the macaroni and transfer them to a baking tray. Pour the tomato sauce and meatballs over the macaroni and mix well to distribute evenly. Add the mozzarella cubes to the top of the macaroni and sprinkle with the grated cheese. Bake for about 15/20 minutes, until the cheese is melted and golden. Remove from the oven and let rest for a few minutes before serving. Sprinkle with fresh chopped parsley before serving.

FETTUCCINE ALFREDO WITH CHICKEN

Preparation time: 10 minutes

Cooking time: 15/20 minutes

Ingredients

(for 4 people):

350 g of fettuccine

300g chicken breast, cut into strips

200 ml of cooking cream

50 g of butter

50 g grated parmesan cheese

Salt and Pepper To Taste

Chopped fresh parsley for garnish

Preparation:

Bring a pot of salted water to the boil and cook the fettuccine according to the package instructions, until al dente. Meanwhile, in a skillet, heat the butter over medium heat. Add the chicken strips to the pan and cook until well browned and cooked through. Reduce the heat to medium-low and add the heavy cream to the pan with the chicken. Mix well and let cook for a few minutes, until the cream is heated. Add the grated cheese to the pan and stir until it has completely melted and a creamy sauce has formed. Season with salt and pepper to taste. Drain the fettuccine and add them to the pan with the alfredo sauce. Mix well to coat the fettuccine with the sauce. Serve the fettuccine alfredo with chicken hot, garnished with fresh chopped parsley.

VEGETABLE MINESTRONE WITH CRISPY BACON

Preparation time: approximately 15 minutes

Cooking time: approximately 25 minutes

Ingredients

(for 4 people):

100 g diced smoked bacon

1 medium onion, finely chopped

2 carrots, diced

2 celery sticks, diced

2 medium potatoes, diced

200g green beans, cut into small pieces

200 g courgettes, cut into cubes

400 g peeled tomatoes, chopped

1 liter of vegetable broth

Salt and pepper to taste. Olive oil to taste

Preparation:

In a large pot, heat a drizzle of olive oil over medium heat. Add the bacon and brown until crispy. Remove the bacon from the pot and set aside. In the same pot, add the onion, carrots and celery. Cook for about 5 minutes or until the vegetables soften slightly. Add the potatoes, green beans, courgettes and chopped peeled tomatoes to the pot. Mix the ingredients well. Pour the vegetable broth into the pan and bring everything to the boil. Then reduce the heat and simmer for about 20/25 minutes, or until all the vegetables are tender. Season with salt and pepper to taste. To serve, spoon the vegetable minestrone into individual bowls and garnish with crispy bacon and freshly chopped parsley.

TORTELLINI IN CHICKEN BROTH

Preparation time: approximately 5 minutes

Cooking time: approximately 10 minutes

Ingredients

(for 4 people):

250 g of tortellini (choice of: meat,

cheese, spinach, etc.)

1 liter of chicken broth

Fresh parsley, chopped (for garnish)

Preparation:

In a large pot, bring the chicken broth to a boil. Add the tortellini to the boiling broth and cook them according to the instructions on the package. It will usually take about 7/10 minutes, but be sure to check the specific instructions on the packaging of the tortellini you have chosen. Once the tortellini are cooked, remove the pan from the heat. To serve, divide the tortellini into individual bowls and pour the hot chicken broth over the top. Garnish with chopped fresh parsley. Preparation and cooking times may vary depending on your cooking experience and the specifications of your stove, so I recommend referring to the instructions on the tortellini packaging to ensure you get precise cooking.

PAPPARDELLE WITH BEEF SAUCE

Preparation time: approximately 15/20 minutes

Ragu cooking time: approximately 1 hour

Ingredients

(for 4 people):

300 g of fresh or dried pappardelle

500g minced beef

1 medium onion, finely chopped

2 cloves garlic, minced

400 g peeled tomatoes, chopped

2 tablespoons of tomato paste

1/2 cup red wine

1 cup beef broth

2 tablespoons olive oil, Salt and pepper to taste

Preparation:

In a large pot, heat the olive oil over medium heat. Add the onion and garlic and let them brown slightly. Add the ground beef to the pot and cook until well browned and fully cooked. Add the tomato paste and mix well with the meat. Cook for a couple of minutes to let the flavors develop. Pour the red wine into the pan and let it evaporate completely. Add the chopped peeled tomatoes and the meat broth. Mix well, bring to the boil, then reduce the heat and simmer for at least an hour, stirring occasionally. If the ragout dries out too much during cooking, you can add a little water or broth. In the meantime, cook the pappardelle in plenty of salted water following the instructions on the package. Drain them al dente. Drain the pappardelle and add them directly to the pot with the beef ragù. Mix well to blend the flavors. Serve the pappardelle with beef ragù hot, garnished with grated cheese and chopped fresh parsley.

ONION SOUP GRATINATED WITH CHEESE

Preparation time: approximately 15 minutes

Soup cooking time: approximately 15 minutes

Ingredients

(for 4 people):

4 large onions, cut into thin slices

2 tablespoons butter

1 liter vegetable broth or chicken broth

2 slices of toasted bread

Grated cheese (e.g

Gruyère or Emmental) to taste

Salt and Pepper To Taste

Preparation:

In a large saucepan, melt the butter over medium heat. Add the onion slices and cook over a low heat, stirring occasionally, until the onions are well caramelized and soft. This takes approximately 30/40 minutes. Add the vegetable broth or chicken broth to the pot with the caramelized onions. Bring to the boil, then reduce the heat and simmer for a further 15 minutes. Meanwhile, preheat the oven grill. Place a slice of toast in each heatproof bowl. Pour the hot onion soup over the toasted bread slices, spreading evenly. Sprinkle grated cheese liberally over the surface of each bowl of soup. Place the bowls under the oven grill and grill until the cheese is melted and golden. Serve the onion soup au gratin hot.

TAGLIOLINI WITH PORCINI MUSHROOMS AND BACON

Preparation time: approximately 15/20 minutes

Cooking time: approximately 20/25 minutes

Ingredients

(for 4 people):

320 g of tagliolini

200 g fresh porcini mushrooms, sliced

100g smoked bacon, diced

2 cloves garlic, finely chopped

1/2 cup vegetable broth

1/2 cup fresh cream

1/4 cup dry white wine

2 tablespoons olive oil, Salt and pepper to taste

Fresh parsley, chopped (for garnish)

Preparation:

In a large skillet, heat the olive oil over medium heat. Add the bacon and brown until crispy. Remove the bacon from the pan and set aside. In the same pan, add the garlic cloves and sliced porcini mushrooms. Cook for about 5 minutes or until the mushrooms soften and release their liquid. Add the white wine to the pan and let it evaporate for a few minutes. Add the vegetable broth and fresh cream to the pan. Mix the ingredients well and cook over medium-low heat for about 10/15 minutes, until the liquid reduces slightly and thickens. In the meantime, cook the tagliolini in plenty of salted water following the instructions on the package. Drain them al dente. Add the drained tagliolini to the pan with the mushrooms and cream sauce. Season with salt and pepper to taste. Mix well to blend the flavors. Serve the tagliolini with hot porcini mushrooms and bacon.

CHICKEN CANNELLONI WITH SPINACH AND RICOTTA

Preparation time: approximately 30 minutes

Cooking time: approximately 40/45 minutes

Ingredients

(for 4 people):

12 dried or fresh cannelloni

300g cooked chicken breast, finely chopped

200 g of fresh spinach, boiled and squeezed

250 g of ricotta, 1 egg

1/2 cup tomato sauce

1/2 cup of bechamel

100 g grated Parmesan cheese

Salt and pepper to taste, Olive oil to taste

Preparation:

Preheat the oven to 180°C. In a bowl, mix the minced chicken, the boiled and squeezed spinach, the ricotta, the egg, half the grated cheese, salt and pepper. Mix well until a homogeneous mixture is obtained. Fill the cannelloni with the chicken, spinach and ricotta mixture using a teaspoon or pastry bag. In a baking pan, spread a thin layer of tomato sauce on the bottom. Place the cannelloni filled with tomato sauce on the baking tray. Pour the béchamel sauce evenly over the cannelloni. Sprinkle the remaining grated cheese over the béchamel. Cover the pan with foil and bake in the oven for about 30 minutes. Next, remove the foil and cook for a further 10 to 15 minutes or until the cannelloni are golden brown and the cheese has melted. Remove the chicken cannelloni with spinach and ricotta from the oven and let them rest for a few minutes before serving.

BOSCAIOLA BUTTERFLIES WITH SAUSAGE

Preparation time: 10 minutes

Cooking times: 40 minutes

Doses for 4 people:

Ingredients:

350 g of farfalle

250 g of fresh sausage, skinless and crumbled

1 onion, finely chopped

200 g button mushrooms, sliced

200 ml of fresh cream

1/2 cup beef broth

Salt and Pepper To Taste

Fresh parsley, chopped (for garnish)

Preparation:

Cook the farfalle in plenty of water

salted according to the instructions on the package. Drain them al dente and set them aside. In a pan, cook the crumbled sausage until it is golden brown. Remove it from the pan and set it aside. In the same pan, add the chopped onion and sliced mushrooms. Cook until the vegetables soften and release their liquid. Add the previously cooked sausage to the pan with the vegetables. Mix well. Add the white wine (if desired) and let it evaporate for a few minutes. Add the cream and beef broth to the pan. Mix well, bring to the boil, then reduce the heat and simmer for about 1015 minutes, until the sauce thickens slightly. Season with salt and pepper to taste. Add the farfalle to the pan with the sauce and mix well to combine with the ingredients. Serve the farfalle alla Boscaiola hot, garnished with fresh chopped parsley.

TOMATO SOUP WITH CRISPY HAM

Preparation times: 10/15 minutes

Cooking times: 20/25 minutes

Doses for 4 people:, Ingredients:

800 g of peeled tomatoes

1 onion, finely chopped

2 cloves garlic, finely chopped

4 slices of raw ham

500 ml of vegetable broth

2 tablespoons olive oil Salt and pepper to taste

Fresh basil, chopped (for garnish)

Preparation:

In a saucepan, heat the olive oil over medium heat. Add the chopped onion and minced garlic. Cook until they become

soft and translucent. Add the peeled tomatoes to the pot, mashing them with a fork or wooden spoon to break them into smaller pieces. Add vegetable broth or chicken broth to the pot. Bring to the boil, then reduce the heat and simmer for about 2025 minutes to develop the flavours. Meanwhile, preheat the oven grill. Place the ham slices on a baking tray lined with baking paper. Place the pan under the grill and cook the ham until crispy. Remove the crispy ham from the oven and let it cool slightly. Crumble it or cut it into small pieces. Using an immersion blender or traditional blender, blend the tomato soup until smooth. Season with salt and pepper to taste. Serve the tomato soup hot, garnished with crumbled crispy ham and chopped fresh basil.

CHICKEN AND VEGETABLE LASAGNE

Preparation time: 30 minutes

Cooking Times: 45 minutes

Doses for 4 people:

Ingredients:

250g lasagne sheets

400g chicken breast, cooked and shredded

1 courgette, diced

1 red pepper, diced

1 onion, finely chopped

2 cloves garlic, finely chopped

400 g of tomato sauce

200 g of grated cheese

Olive oil to taste Salt and pepper to taste

Fresh basil for garnish (optional)

Preparation:

Preheat the oven to 180°C. In a pot, cook the lasagna following the instructions on the package. Drain them and keep them aside. In a pan, heat some olive oil and add the chopped onion and garlic. Fry them until they become translucent. Add the courgette and pepper to the pan and cook for a few minutes, until the vegetables soften slightly. Add the shredded chicken breast to the pan and mix well. Season with salt and pepper to taste. Cook for another 23 minutes. Add the tomato sauce to the pan and mix well. Leave to cook for about 5 minutes, so that the flavors blend. In a baking pan, spread a thin layer of tomato sauce on the bottom.

Add a layer of lasagna sheets, then a layer of the chicken and vegetable filling. Continue alternating layers until you run out of ingredients, finishing with a layer of lasagna. Sprinkle the grated cheese over the surface of the lasagna. Cover the pan with foil and bake in a preheated oven for about 30/35 minutes. Next, uncover the pan and cook for another 10 minutes, until the cheese on the surface is golden and the lasagne is well cooked. Once ready, let the lasagna rest for a few minutes. Garnish with fresh basil if desired and serve hot.

PILOT RICE WITH SAUSAGE

Preparation time: 15 minutes

Cooking times: 25/30 minutes

Doses for 4 people:

Ingredients:

300 g of Arborio or Carnaroli rice

200 g of sausage, peeled and crumbled

1 onion, finely chopped

2 cloves garlic, finely chopped

1 carrot, diced

1 stalk celery, diced

400 g of tomato sauce

1 liter of vegetable broth

Olive oil to taste Salt and pepper to taste

Preparation:

In a large pot, heat some olive oil. Add the onion, garlic, chopped carrot and celery and fry until the vegetables soften. Add the crumbled sausage to the pan and cook until golden brown. Add the rice to the pan and toast it lightly for a few minutes, stirring constantly. Add the tomato sauce and mix well. Leave to cook for a couple of minutes, so that the rice absorbs the flavors. Gradually add the hot vegetable broth, one ladle at a time, stirring constantly. Wait for the rice to absorb the broth before adding more. Continue cooking the rice, adding broth and stirring, until the rice is cooked al dente and has absorbed the liquid (about 1520 minutes). Taste and adjust salt and pepper to taste. Once the rice is cooked and creamy, remove it from the heat and let it rest for a few minutes. Garnish the pilot rice with chopped fresh parsley if desired and serve hot.

LINGUINE WITH CLAMS AND BACON

Preparation time: 30 minutes

Cooking times: 20/2 5 minutes

Ingredients:

Doses for 4 people:

500 g of linguine

1 kg of fresh clams

100 g of smoked bacon

Garlic (2 cloves)

Red chili pepper (to taste)

Olive oil (2 tablespoons)

Chopped fresh parsley (to taste)

Salt and Pepper To Taste)

Preparation:

Clean and open the clams, eliminating those already open or broken. Cook the linguine in plenty of salted water until al dente. In a pan, heat the olive oil and add the minced garlic and red chilli for flavour. Add the diced smoked bacon to the pan and brown it. Add the clams to the pan and cover with a lid to open over medium-high heat. Drain the linguine and add it to the pan with the clams and bacon. Season with salt and pepper to taste and mix gently. Sprinkle with fresh chopped parsley and serve hot.

SORRENTINA GNOCCHI WITH COOKED HAM

Preparation time: 25 minutes

Cooking times: 20/25 minutes

Ingredients:

Doses for 4 people:

500 g of gnocchi

400 g of tomato pulp

150 g of mozzarella

100 g of cooked ham

1 clove of garlic

Fresh basil (to taste)

Olive oil (2 tablespoons)

Salt and Pepper To Taste)

Preparation:

In a pan, bring salted water to the boil to cook the gnocchi. In a pan, heat the olive oil and add the chopped garlic clove for flavour. Add the tomato pulp to the pan and cook over medium-low heat for 20/25 minutes to obtain a thick sauce. Add the diced cooked ham to the tomato sauce and mix. Cook the gnocchi in boiling salted water until they rise to the surface. Drain the gnocchi and add them to the pan with the tomato sauce and cooked ham. Add the diced mozzarella to the pan and mix gently. Season with salt and pepper to taste and garnish with fresh basil. Serve hot.

BLACK BEAN SOUP WITH CHORIZO

Preparation time: 15 minutes

(+ Soaking the beans: 8 hours)

Cooking times: 1 hour

ingredients

Doses for 4 people:

250 g of dried black beans

(or 500g canned black beans)

200 g of smoked chorizo

1 onion, 2 cloves of garlic

2 carrots, 2 stalks of celery

1 bay leaf

Vegetable broth (about 1 liter)

Olive oil, Salt and pepper (to taste)

Chopped fresh parsley (for garnish)

Preparation:

If using dried beans, soak in cold water for at least 8 hours or according to package instructions. Drain and rinse. In a large pot, heat some olive oil and add the chopped onion, garlic, carrots and celery. Fry for a few minutes. Add the black beans to the pot and cover them with vegetable broth. Add the bay leaf and bring everything to the boil. Reduce heat and simmer for 12 hours (or according to the directions on the dried bean package) until the beans are soft and tender. In the meantime, cut the chorizo into thin slices and brown in a non-stick pan for 10/15 minutes or until crispy. Add the chorizo to the bean soup and mix gently. Season with salt and pepper according to taste. Serve the black bean soup with a sprinkle of chopped fresh parsley on top.

RISOTTO WITH PORCINI MUSHROOMS

Preparation time: 20 minutes

Cooking times: 35 minutes

Cooking of porcini mushrooms: 10/12 minutes

Ingredients:

Doses for 4 people:

320 g of Arborio or Carnaroli rice

200 g of fresh porcini mushrooms

(40 g dried porcini mushrooms, soaked)

1 onion, 2 cloves of garlic

1 liter of hot vegetable broth

100 ml of dry white wine

Grated Parmesan (to taste)

Butter (30 g), Olive oil

Salt and Pepper To Taste)

Chopped fresh parsley (for garnish)

Preparation:

If using dried porcini mushrooms, soak in hot water for about 2030 minutes. Drain them and squeeze them well. If using fresh porcini mushrooms, clean and slice them. In a large pot, heat some olive oil and add the chopped onion and garlic. Fry for a few minutes until the onion becomes transparent. Add the rice to the pan and toast it lightly for a couple of minutes, stirring constantly. Add the white wine and let it evaporate completely.

Gradually add the hot vegetable broth, one ladle at a time, stirring constantly and waiting for the liquid to be absorbed before adding more. Meanwhile, in a separate pan, heat some olive oil and add the porcini mushrooms. Cook them for 10/12 minutes or until they are soft and golden. Season with salt and pepper. Continue adding the vegetable broth to the risotto and stirring until the rice is al dente and the consistency of the risotto is creamy. Turn off the heat and add the butter and grated Parmesan to the risotto. Stir until the butter has melted and the cheese is combined. Cover the risotto and let it rest for a few minutes. Serve the porcini mushroom risotto garnished with chopped fresh parsley on top.

FUSILLI WITH MEAT SAUCE

Preparation time: 15 minutes

Cooking times: 72 minutes

Ingredients

for 4 people:

400 g of fusilli

400 g of minced beef

1 onion, 2 cloves of garlic

400 g of tomato puree

1 can of peeled tomatoes, 1 carrot

1 stalk of celery

Olive oil, Salt and pepper (to taste)

Chopped fresh parsley (for garnish)

Preparation:

In a large pot, heat some olive oil and add the chopped onion, garlic, carrot and celery. Fry for a few minutes until the vegetables become soft. Add the minced meat to the pan and sauté until well cooked and browned. Add the tomato puree and the crushed peeled tomatoes to the pan. Mix well. Cover the pan and simmer for 12 hours, stirring occasionally, until the sauce has reduced and thickened. In the meantime, cook the fusilli in plenty of salted water until they are al dente. Drain them and keep aside. Add the fusilli to the pan with the meat sauce and mix well. Season with salt and pepper to taste. Serve the fusilli with meat sauce hot, sprinkled with fresh chopped parsley.

TORTELLINI WITH BACON AND CREAM

Preparation time: 15 minutes

Cooking times: 57 minutes

Ingredients

for 4 people:

500 g of tortellini (filled to taste)

150 g of smoked bacon

200 ml of cooking cream

1 onion

2 cloves of garlic

Olive oil

Salt and Pepper To Taste)

Preparation:

In a large pot, bring the water for cooking the tortellini to the boil.

Cook the tortellini according to the instructions on the package. Drain them and keep aside. In a pan, heat some olive oil and add the diced smoked bacon. Fry it until it is crispy and golden. Add the chopped onion and garlic to the pan with the bacon and fry for a few minutes until soft. Add the cooking cream to the pan and mix well. Cook over medium-low heat for a few minutes until the sauce has heated through and thickened slightly. Add the tortellini to the pan with the bacon and cream sauce. Stir gently to coat the tortellini with the sauce. Season with salt and pepper to taste. Serve the tortellini with hot bacon and cream, sprinkled with fresh chopped parsley.

PAPPARDELLE WITH RABBIT SAUCE

Preparation time: 20 minutes

Cooking of the rabbit ragout: 23 hours

Cooking pappardelle: 810 minutes

Ingredients

for 4 people:

400 g of pappardelle

600 g of boneless rabbit meat

1 onion, 2 carrots

2 sticks of celery, 2 cloves of garlic

400 g of tomato puree

250 ml of red wine

Vegetable broth (about 500 ml)

Olive oil, Salt and pepper (to taste)

Preparation:

In a large pot, heat some olive oil and add the onion, carrots and chopped celery. Fry for a few minutes until the vegetables become soft. Add the rabbit meat to the pan and brown until golden on all sides. Add the chopped garlic and fry for a minute. Add the red wine to the pan and let it evaporate for a few minutes. Add the tomato puree and enough vegetable broth to cover the rabbit meat. Mix well. Cover the pot and simmer for 23 hours, stirring occasionally, until the rabbit meat is tender and shreds easily. In the meantime, cook the pappardelle in plenty of salted water until al dente. Drain them and keep aside. Flake the rabbit meat with two forks and add it to the ragù. Mix well and cook for another 1015 minutes. Season with salt and pepper according to taste. Serve the pappardelle with rabbit ragù hot, sprinkled with fresh chopped parsley.

CHICKEN SOUP WITH VEGETABLES AND COUSCOUS

Preparation time: 20 minutes

Cooking times: 30/40 minutes

Ingredients

for 4 people:

4 chicken thighs

1 onion, 2 carrots

2 sticks of celery

2 potatoes, 2 courgettes

1 red pepper

2 cloves of garlic

1 liter of chicken broth

200 g of couscous

Olive oil, Salt and pepper (to taste)

Preparation:

In a large pot, heat a little olive oil and add the diced onion, carrots, celery, potatoes, courgettes and pepper. Sauté for a few minutes until the vegetables begin to soften. Add the chicken thighs to the pot and sauté until lightly browned. Add the chopped garlic and fry for a minute. Pour the chicken broth into the pot and bring to a boil. Reduce the heat and cook over medium-low heat for 30/40 minutes, until the chicken is well cooked and the vegetables are tender. Meanwhile, prepare the couscous according to the package instructions. Drain the chicken and shred it with two forks. Add the shredded chicken to the chicken and vegetable soup. Season the soup with salt and pepper to taste. Serve the chicken soup with vegetables hot, accompanied by couscous.

TAGLIATELLE WITH LAMB SAUCE

Preparation time: 20 minutes

Cooking of the lamb ragout: 2/3 hours

Cooking of tagliatelle: 10 minutes

Ingredients

for 4 people:

400 g of tagliatelle

600 g of lamb cut into cubes

1 onion, 2 carrots 2 sticks of celery

2 cloves of garlic 400 g of tomato puree 250 ml of red wine

Vegetable broth (about 500 ml)

Olive oil, Salt and pepper (to taste)

Preparation:

In a large pot, heat some olive oil and add the onion, carrots and chopped celery. Fry for a few minutes until the vegetables become soft. Add the lamb to the pot and brown until browned on all sides. Add the chopped garlic and fry for a minute. Add the red wine to the pan and let it evaporate for a few minutes. Add the tomato puree and enough vegetable stock to cover the lamb. Mix well. Cover the pot and simmer for 23 hours, stirring occasionally, until the lamb is tender and shreds easily. In the meantime, cook the tagliatelle in abundant salted water until they are al dente. Drain them and keep aside. Tear the lamb apart with two forks and add it to the ragù. Mix well and cook for another 10/15 minutes. Season with salt and pepper according to taste. Serve the tagliatelle with lamb ragout hot, sprinkled with fresh chopped parsley.

PASTA AND BEANS WITH BACON

Preparation time: 20 minutes

Cooking times: 30/40 minutes

Ingredients

for 4 people:

250 g of short pasta

200 g of smoked bacon,

cut into cubes, 1 onion

2 cloves of garlic, 2 carrots

2 sticks of celery

400 g of cannellini beans in

can (rinsed and drained)

800 ml of vegetable broth

400 g of tomato puree

Olive oil, Salt and pepper (to taste)

Preparation:

In a large pot, heat some olive oil and add the smoked bacon. Fry it until it is crispy and golden. Add the chopped onion, garlic, carrots and celery to the pot. Fry for a few minutes until the vegetables become soft. Add the tomato puree, cannellini beans and vegetable broth to the pot. Mix well. Bring the soup to the boil, reduce the heat and cook over medium-low heat for 20 to 30 minutes, until the vegetables are tender and the flavors have blended. Meanwhile, cook the pasta in plenty of salted water until al dente. Drain it and keep it aside. Add the pasta to the pot with the bean soup and mix well. Season with salt and pepper to taste. Serve the pasta and beans with hot bacon, sprinkled with fresh chopped parsley on top.

HAM AND CHEESE RAVIOLI WITH BUTTER AND SAGE

Preparation times: approximately 30 minutes

Cooking times: approximately 10/12 minutes

Doses for 4 people

Ingredients:

250 g ravioli pasta

(preferably fresh)

100 g of raw ham

100 g of cheese

(mozzarella or cream cheese)

50 g of butter, 68 sage leaves

Salt and Pepper To Taste

Preparation:

Cut the ham into small cubes and chop the cheese. Roll out the ravioli dough on a floured surface. Place a teaspoon of ham and cheese on half of the pasta, leaving enough space between the fillings. Fold the other half of the pastry over the filling and press the edges with your fingers to seal. Bring a pan of salted water to the boil and cook the ravioli until they rise to the surface (about 10/12 minutes). Meanwhile, in a skillet, melt the butter over medium-high heat until it begins to brown slightly. Add the sage leaves and let them cook for a few seconds until they become crispy. Drain the cooked ravioli and transfer them to the pan with the butter and sage. Gently mix the ravioli to flavor them with the butter and sage. Add salt and pepper if necessary. Serve the ravioli hot and garnish with a few crispy sage leaves.

SPINACH LASAGNA WITH BECHAMELLE AND BACON

Preparation times: approximately 30 minutes

Cooking times: approximately 40/45 minutes

Doses for 4 people

Ingredients:

250 g of egg lasagne

300 g of fresh spinach

200 g of smoked bacon

500 ml of bechamel

100 g of grated parmesan

Olive oil to taste Salt and pepper to taste

Preparation:

Preheat the oven to 180°C. Boil the spinach in boiling salted water for a few minutes, then drain them and squeeze them to remove excess water. Cut the bacon into cubes and brown it in a pan with a drizzle of olive oil until it becomes crispy. Remove the bacon from the pan and set aside. In a baking pan, spread a thin layer of béchamel on the bottom. Arrange a layer of lasagna, then cover with a layer of spinach and bacon. Add some grated cheese and bechamel. Repeat the previous steps until you run out of ingredients, finishing with a layer of béchamel sauce and grated cheese. Cover the pan with foil and bake for about 30 minutes. Remove the foil and continue cooking for another 10/15 minutes, or until the surface of the lasagne is golden and crispy. Remove the lasagna from the oven and let it rest for a few minutes before serving. Cut into portions and serve hot.

SPAGHETTI PUTTANESCA WITH ANCHOVIES AND OLIVES

Preparation times: approximately 10 minutes

Cooking times: approximately 15/20 minutes

Doses for 4 people

Ingredients:

320 g of spaghetti

4 anchovy fillets in oil

2 cloves garlic, minced

400 g peeled tomatoes, crushed

60 g of black olives, pitted and cut

2 tablespoons capers, rinsed

Dried red chili pepper, chopped

Extra virgin olive oil to taste

Salt to taste

Preparation:

Bring a pot of salted water to a boil and cook the spaghetti according to package instructions until al dente. In a pan, heat some olive oil and add the minced garlic and dried red chili pepper (if desired). Fry for a few minutes until the garlic turns golden. Add the anchovy fillets in oil to the pan and let them melt. Add the crushed peeled tomatoes, the sliced olives and the capers. Mix well. Let the sauce cook over medium heat for about 10 minutes, until it thickens slightly. Drain the spaghetti al dente and transfer them to the pan with the sauce. Mix well to mix the ingredients. Add salt if necessary. Serve the spaghetti puttanesca hot.

BEEF CANNELLONI
WITH TOMATO SAUCE

Preparation times: approximately 30 minutes

Cooking times: approximately 50 minutes

Doses for 4 people

Ingredients:

12 cannelloni

400g minced beef

1 onion, finely chopped

2 cloves garlic, minced

400 g of tomato sauce

200 g of ricotta

100 g of grated parmesan

Olive oil to taste

Salt and Pepper To Taste

Preparation:

Preheat the oven to 180°C. In a pan, heat some olive oil and add the chopped onion and garlic. Fry them until they turn golden. Add the ground beef to the skillet and cook until browned and fully cooked. Add the tomato sauce to the pan and mix well with the ground meat. Let it cook for a few minutes. In a separate bowl, mix the ricotta with half the grated cheese. Season with salt and pepper. Fill the cannelloni with the ground meat mixture and place them on a lightly greased baking tray. Pour the remaining tomato sauce over the cannelloni, covering them completely.

Sprinkle the surface with the remaining grated cheese. Cover the pan with foil and bake for about 30 minutes. Remove the foil and continue cooking for another 15/20 minutes, or until the cannelloni are well cooked and the surface is golden. Remove the cannelloni from the oven and let them rest for a few minutes before serving. Serve the cannelloni hot and garnish with some chopped fresh parsley, if desired.

BUTTERFLIES WITH OF SAUSAGE AND MUSHROOMS SAUCE

Preparation times: approximately 10 minutes

Cooking times: approximately 20/25 minutes

Doses for 4 people

Ingredients:

320 g farfalle pasta

300 g of fresh sausage, peeled and crumbled

200 g button mushrooms, sliced

1 onion, finely chopped

2 cloves garlic, minced

400 g of tomato puree

120 ml of dry white wine

Extra virgin olive oil to taste

Salt and Pepper To Taste

Preparation:

Bring a pot of salted water to boil and cook farfalle according to package instructions until al dente. In a pan, heat some olive oil and add the chopped onion and garlic. Fry them until they turn golden. Add the crumbled sausage to the pan and cook until well browned. Add the sliced mushrooms and continue to cook for a few minutes until the mushrooms soften. Pour the white wine into the pan and let it evaporate completely. Add the tomato puree and mix well. Let the sauce cook over medium-low heat for about 10/15 minutes, or until it thickens slightly. Add salt and pepper to your taste. Drain the farfalle al dente and transfer to the pan with the sauce. Stir gently to combine the ingredients. Serve farfalle with hot sausage and mushroom sauce.

PEAS SOUP WITH HAM

Preparation times: approximately 10 minutes

Cooking times: approximately 25/30 minutes

Doses for 4 people

Ingredients:

400 g of fresh or frozen peas

100 g of raw ham, cut into cubes

1 onion, finely chopped

2 cloves garlic, minced

1 liter of vegetable broth

Extra virgin olive oil to taste

Salt and Pepper To Taste

Preparation:

In a saucepan, heat some olive oil and add the chopped onion and garlic. Fry them until they turn golden. Add the diced raw ham and cook it for a few minutes until it becomes crispy. Add the peas and mix well with the ham and onion. Pour the vegetable broth into the pot and bring to the boil. Reduce the heat and let the soup cook over medium-low heat for about 20/25 minutes, or until the peas are tender. Partially blend the soup with an immersion blender for a creamier consistency (you can leave some peas whole for a more rustic texture, if you prefer). Add salt and pepper to your taste. Serve the ham pea soup hot and garnish with some additional crispy ham, if desired.

RISOTTO WITH TRUFFLE CREAM AND BACON

Preparation times: approximately 10 minutes

Cooking times: approximately 20/25 minutes

Doses for 4 people

Ingredients:

320 g of Arborio or Carnaroli rice

60 g smoked bacon, diced

1 onion, finely chopped

2 cloves garlic, minced

500 ml of vegetable broth

60 ml of dry white wine

2 tablespoons of truffle cream

50 g of grated cheese (parmesan or pecorino)

Extra virgin olive oil to taste. Salt and pepper to taste

Preparation:

In a pan, heat some olive oil and add the diced smoked bacon. Cook it until it becomes crispy. Add the chopped onion and garlic to the pot and sauté until golden brown. Add the rice to the pan and toast it for a few minutes, stirring constantly. Pour the white wine into the pan and let it evaporate completely. Gradually add the vegetable broth to the pot, one ladle at a time, stirring constantly and adding more broth only when the previous one has been absorbed. Continue to cook the risotto, stirring frequently, until the rice is al dente and has reached a creamy consistency. Add the truffle cream to the risotto and mix well. Add salt and pepper to your taste. Add the grated cheese to the risotto and stir until melted and combined well. Serve the risotto with truffle cream and bacon hot.

RECIPES
SECOND DISHES

BAKED CHICKEN WITH AROMATIC SPICES

Preparation times: approximately 1015 minutes

Cooking times: approximately 4050 minutes

Doses for 46 people

Ingredients:

1 whole chicken (about 1.52 kg),

clean and gutted

Aromatic spices to taste

(cumin, oregano, thyme, rosemary)

Salt and Pepper To Taste

Extra virgin olive oil

Lemon juice (optional)

Preparation:

Preheat the oven to 200°C. In a bowl, mix aromatic spices, salt and pepper to create a seasoning blend. Rub the chicken with a little extra virgin olive oil all over the surface. Sprinkle the seasoning mixture all over the surface of the chicken, massaging well to help the spices adhere. You can also sprinkle a little lemon juice on the surface of the chicken for a touch of freshness (optional). Place the chicken on a baking tray and bake in the preheated oven. Cook the chicken for about 4050 minutes, or until the skin is golden and crispy and the meat is cooked through (make sure the internal juices are clear and the internal temperature reaches at least 75°C). Once cooked, remove the chicken from the oven and let it rest for a few minutes before slicing. Slice the chicken and serve hot.

GRILLED BEEF STEAK

Preparation times: approximately 10 minutes

Cooking times: 46 minutes for a steak

Doses for 4 people

Ingredients:

4 beef steaks

(ribeye cut, striploin)

Coarse salt

Freshly ground black pepper

Extra virgin olive oil

Preparation:

Preheat grill to high heat. Before cooking the steak, make sure it is at room temperature. Let it rest outside the refrigerator for about 30 minutes.

Rub the steak with a little extra virgin olive oil on both sides. Season the steak with coarse salt and freshly ground black pepper on both sides, pressing lightly to help the spices adhere to the meat. Place the steak on the preheated grill and cook over high heat for the desired amount of time for your preferred doneness. You can turn the steak halfway through cooking to get an even grill on both sides. Once you reach your desired doneness, transfer the steak to a cutting board and let it rest for a few minutes before serving. This allows the juices to distribute evenly throughout the meat. Cut the steak into slices and serve hot. You can garnish with a drizzle of extra virgin olive oil, if desired.

BARBECUE PORK CHOPS

Preparation times: approximately 15 minutes

Cooking times: approximately 20/25 minutes

Doses for 4 people

Ingredients:

1 kg of pork chops

Barbecue sauce

Salt and Pepper To Taste

Extra virgin olive oil

Preparation:

Preheat grill to medium-high heat. Rub the pork chops with salt and pepper on both sides. Brush both sides of the ribs with the barbecue sauce, covering them well.

Let the ribs marinate for at least 15/20 minutes to absorb the flavors. Brush the grill with a little extra virgin olive oil to prevent the ribs from sticking. Place the pork chops on the preheated grill and cook for approximately 10/12 minutes per side, or until they reach an internal temperature of at least 70/75°F. While cooking, brush the ribs with the remaining barbecue sauce halfway through cooking and turn to cook evenly. Once cooked, remove the ribs from the grill and let them rest for a few minutes before serving. Serve the barbecue pork ribs hot, with additional barbecue sauce if desired.

GRILLED SAUSAGES WITH CARAMELIZED ONIONS

Preparation times: approximately 15 minutes

Cooking times: approximately 20 minutes

Doses for 4 people

Ingredients:

8 Sausages (choose the type

of sausages you prefer)

2 Onions (preferably red or sweet onions), sliced

Brown sugar to taste

Salt and Pepper To Taste

Extra virgin olive oil

Preparation:

Preheat grill to medium-high heat. In a pan, heat some extra virgin olive oil and add the sliced onions. Cook it over medium-low heat,

stirring occasionally, until onions soften and begin to caramelize (about 15 minutes). Add a teaspoon of brown sugar to the caramelized onions and mix well to caramelize them further. Continue cooking for another 12 minutes, until the onions are a nice golden color. Remove from heat and set aside. Brush the grill with a little extra virgin olive oil to prevent the sausages from sticking. Place the sausages on the preheated grill and cook for about 20 minutes, turning occasionally to cook evenly, until they are cooked through and the skin is crispy. During the last 5 minutes of cooking, you can brush the sausages with a little extra virgin olive oil to make them even more succulent. Once cooked, remove the sausages to the grill and let them rest for a few minutes. Serve the grilled sausages hot, accompanied by caramelized onions as a side dish.

ROAST VEAL WITH MUSHROOM SAUCE

Preparation times: approximately 20 minutes

Cooking times: approximately 1 hour

Doses for 4 people

Ingredients:

1 kg of veal (side, thigh or shoulder)

Salt and pepper to taste Extra virgin olive oil

200 g of mixed mushrooms

(champignons, porcini mushrooms, etc.)

1 onion, finely chopped

2 cloves garlic, finely chopped

200 ml of meat broth

200 ml of cooking cream

Preparation:

Preheat the oven to 180°C. Rub the veal with salt and pepper on all sides. Warm up an ovenproof pan with a little extra virgin olive oil. Brown the veal on all sides until it takes on a nice golden colour. Transfer the veal to a baking tray and cook in a preheated oven for about 1 hour, or until the internal temperature reaches 65/70°C for medium rare. Meanwhile, prepare the mushroom sauce. In a separate pan, heat some extra virgin olive oil and add the chopped onion and garlic. Cook until soft and translucent. Add the mushrooms to the pan and cook until golden and soft. Add the meat broth and let it cook for a few minutes, then add the cooking cream and mix well. Let the sauce simmer over medium-low heat until it thickens slightly. Once the veal roast is cooked, remove from the oven and let rest for a few minutes before slicing. Serve the sliced veal roast with the mushroom sauce on top and garnish with chopped fresh parsley, if desired.

LAMB CHOPS WITH MINT

Preparation times: 15/20 minutes

Cooking times: 10/15 minutes

Doses for 4 people

Ingredients:

4 lamb chops

Salt and Pepper To Taste

Extra virgin olive oil

Lemon juice

Fresh mint, finely chopped

Preparation:

Rub the lamb chops with salt, pepper, a little extra virgin olive oil and a few drops of lemon juice on both sides.

Sprinkle chopped fresh mint over lamb chops, pressing lightly to adhere. Let the lamb chops marinate in the refrigerator for at least 30 minutes, so that the flavors blend. Heat a heatproof pan or grill and brush a little extra virgin olive oil. Cook the lamb chops on the preheated pan or grill over medium-high heat for about 4 to 6 minutes per side, or until cooked to your preferred doneness. Once cooked, remove the lamb chops from the pan or grill and let them rest for a few minutes before serving. Serve hot minted lamb chops as a main course.

BEEF BURGER WITH MELTED CHEESE

Preparation times: approximately 15/20 minutes

Cooking times: approximately 10/15 minutes

Doses for 4 people

Ingredients:

500g minced beef

Salt and Pepper To Taste

Sliced cheese

Bread for hamburgers

Condiments of your choice (lettuce, tomato, onion, pickles, mayonnaise, ketchup)

Preparation:

In a bowl, mix the ground beef with salt and pepper to your taste.

You can also add other spices or flavors of your choice. Divide the meat into 4 equal portions and shape burgers with your hands, compacting the meat slightly. Heat a pan or grill over medium-high heat and brush on a little extra virgin olive oil. Cook the burgers on the preheated pan or grill for about 4 to 6 minutes per side, or until they reach the desired doneness. During the last minutes of cooking, add a slice of cheese over the meatballs and cover with a lid to melt. Lightly toast the hamburger bun on the same pan or grill. Assemble the burgers, placing each beef patty with melted cheese inside the burger bun, and add toppings of your choice. Serve the beef burgers with melted cheese hot and accompany them with fries or salad, if desired.

GRILLED TUNA STEAK

Preparation times: approximately 10/15 minutes

Cooking times: approximately 3/5 minutes per side

Doses for 4 people

Ingredients:

4 fresh tuna fillets

Salt and Pepper To Taste

Extra virgin olive oil

Lemon juice (optional)

Fresh herbs (such as thyme,

rosemary, parsley, etc.) optional

Preparation:

Rub the tuna fillets with salt and pepper on both sides. If you want, you can squeeze a little lemon juice over the tuna fillets to add a touch of acidity.

If you wish, you can also add fresh aromatic herbs, such as thyme or rosemary, to flavor the tuna. Leave the tuna to marinate for about 10/15 minutes to absorb the flavours. Heat a non-stick griddle or pan over medium-high heat and brush a little extra virgin olive oil. Cook the tuna fillets on the preheated griddle or pan for about 35 minutes per side, or until they are well sealed on the outside but remain pink on the inside. The cooking time depends on the thickness of the fillets and the desired degree of doneness. Once cooked, remove the tuna fillets from the plate or pan and let them rest for a few minutes. Serve the grilled tuna steaks hot, cut into thin slices, accompanied by side dishes of your choice such as salad, grilled vegetables or rice.

CHICKEN STUFFED WITH HAM AND CHEESE

Preparation times: approximately 20/30 minutes

Cooking times: approximately 40/50 minutes

Doses for 4 people

Ingredients:

4 boneless, skinless chicken breasts

Salt and Pepper To Taste

Slices of raw ham

Slices of cheese

(such as mozzarella, provolone,)

Extra virgin olive oil

Dried aromatic herbs

(oregano, thyme, rosemary)

Kitchen string or toothpick

Preparation:

Preheat the oven to 180°C. Divide the chicken breasts in half lengthwise, but without completely separating the two sides. Open the chicken breasts and flatten slightly with a meat mallet or the palm of your hand. Season the chicken breasts with salt, pepper and a sprinkle of dried herbs on both sides. Place a slice of ham and a slice of cheese in the center of each open chicken breast. Fold the sides of the chicken breast over the filling, as if to form a roll, and close with a toothpick or tie with kitchen string to keep the filling in place. Heat a non-stick pan with a little extra virgin olive oil and cook the stuffed chicken breasts over medium-high heat for a few minutes to brown all sides.

Transfer the stuffed chicken breasts to a baking tray and cook in the preheated oven for about 30/40 minutes, or until the chicken is cooked completely and the cheese inside is melted and stringy. Once cooked, let the stuffed chicken breasts rest for a few minutes before removing the toothpick or kitchen string. Serve the chicken stuffed with ham and cheese hot, cut into slices, accompanied by side dishes of your choice such as baked potatoes, grilled vegetables or salad.

GRILLED MIXED MEAT SKEWERS

Preparation times: approximately 20/30 minutes

Cooking times: approximately 10/15 minutes

Doses for 4 people

Ingredients:

500 g of mixed beef,

pork, chicken, lamb, cut into cubes

Salt and Pepper To Taste

Extra virgin olive oil

Spices or marinade of your choice (such as paprika,

curry, garlic powder, lemon juice, etc.)

Vegetables of your choice (such as peppers, onions,

cherry tomatoes, courgettes, etc.), cut into cubes

Preparation:

In a bowl, season the mixed meat with salt, pepper, extra virgin olive oil and the spices or marinade of your choice. Leave to marinate for at least 20/30 minutes to absorb the flavours. Prepare the skewers by alternating meat cubes and vegetables on metal or wooden skewers, leaving some space between the pieces for even cooking. Heat the grill or a grill pan over medium-high heat and brush a little extra virgin olive oil. Cook the skewers on the preheated grill or pan for about 5 to 8 minutes per side, or until the meat is cooked through and the vegetables are soft and lightly charred. While cooking, you can brush the skewers with some of the remaining marinade to add flavor and keep them juicy. Once cooked, remove the skewers to the grill or pan and let them rest for a few minutes before serving.

BEEF FILLET WITH GREEN PEPPER SAUCE

Preparation times: approximately 10/15 minutes

Cooking times: approximately 10/15 minutes

Doses for 4 people

Ingredients:

4 beef fillets of approximately 200 g each

Salt and Pepper To Taste

Extra virgin olive oil

2 tablespoons green pepper in

brine, drained and crushed

200 ml of cooking cream

50ml brandy (optional)

Preparation:

Pre Heat a heatproof pan over medium-high heat and brush on a little oil extra virgin olive oil. Season the beef tenderloins with salt and pepper on both sides. Cook the beef fillets on the preheated pan for approximately 3/5 minutes per side, or until they reach the desired degree of doneness. You can adjust the cooking time depending on your cooking preferences (rare, medium rare, well done). Once cooked, transfer the beef fillets to a plate and cover with foil to keep warm. In the same pan, add the pickled green pepper and stir for a few seconds. Add the heavy cream and brandy (if desired) and mix well. Let it cook for a few minutes until the sauce thickens slightly. Add butter (optional) to enrich the sauce and stir until melted. Remove the sauce from the heat and add salt and pepper, if necessary. Serve the beef fillets hot, sliced, with the green pepper sauce on top.

CHICKEN CACCIATORA

Preparation times: approximately 15 minutes

Cooking times: approximately 50 minutes

Doses for 4 people

Ingredients:

6 pieces chicken (such as thighs, breasts, wings)

Salt and Pepper To Taste

Flour to coat the chicken

Extra virgin olive oil

1 large onion, cut into slices

23 cloves garlic, minced

200 ml of tomato puree

200ml chicken broth

1 sprig of rosemary 1 bay leaf

100g black olives, pitted

Preparation:

Season the chicken with salt and pepper on both the sides, then lightly coat it in flour. Heat a heatproof pan over medium-high heat and add a little extra virgin olive oil. Fry the chicken in the preheated skillet until golden brown on both sides. Remove the chicken from the pan and set aside. In the same pan, add the onion and garlic and sauté until soft and translucent. Add the tomato puree, chicken broth, rosemary, bay leaf, and red wine (if desired). Mix well. Return the chicken to the pan and bring everything to a boil. Reduce the heat to medium-low, cover the pan and let cook for about 40 minutes, or until the chicken is tender and fully cooked. Add the black olives and sliced mushrooms (if desired) to the pan and continue cooking for another 5 to 10 minutes. Remove the rosemary sprig and bay leaf before serving. Serve the chicken Cacciatore hot, accompanied by side dishes of your choice such as baked potatoes, rice or vegetables.

LAMB CHOPS WITH ROSEMARY

Preparation times: approximately 15 minutes

Cooking times: approximately 15 minutes

Doses for 4 people

Ingredients:

8 lamb chops

Salt and Pepper To Taste

Extra virgin olive oil

23 sprigs of fresh rosemary

2 cloves garlic, minced

Juice of half a lemon

Preparation:

Preheat a grill or nonstick skillet over medium-high heat. Season the lamb chops with salt and pepper on both sides. Brush a little olive oil on both sides of the chops. Add fresh rosemary and minced garlic to the chops, pressing lightly to adhere. Grill the lamb chops for about 4 to 6 minutes per side, or until they reach the desired doneness. You can adjust the cooking time depending on your cooking preferences (rare, medium rare, well done). While cooking, you can squeeze lemon juice onto the ribs to add a touch of freshness. Once cooked, transfer the lamb chops to a plate and let them rest for a few minutes before serving. Serve the rosemary lamb chops hot, accompanied by side dishes of your choice such as roast potatoes, grilled vegetables or salad.

HORSE STEAK WITH GARLIC SAUCE

Preparation times: approximately 10/15 minutes

Cooking times: approximately 10/15 minutes

Doses for 4 people

Ingredients:

4 horse steaks

Salt and Pepper To Taste

Extra virgin olive oil

46 cloves garlic, minced

Fresh parsley, chopped

Lemon juice

Preparation:

Preheat a grill or nonstick skillet over medium-high heat.

Season the horse steaks with salt and pepper on both sides. Brush a little olive oil on both sides of the steaks. Add the minced garlic to the steaks and press lightly to adhere. Grill the horse steaks for about 46 minutes per side, or until they reach the desired doneness. You can adjust the cooking time depending on your cooking preferences (rare, medium rare, well done). While cooking, you can squeeze a little lemon juice onto the steaks to add freshness. Once cooked, transfer the horse steaks to a plate and let them rest for a few minutes before serving. Sprinkle chopped parsley over the steaks just before serving. Serve the horse steaks with garlic sauce hot, accompanied by your choice of side dishes such as baked potatoes, grilled vegetables or salad.

ROAST PORK WITH BAKED POTATOES

Preparation times: approximately 15/20 minutes

Cooking times: approximately 1 hour and 30 minutes

Doses for 4 people

Ingredients:

1 kg of roast pork

Salt and Pepper To Taste

Aromatic herbs (rosemary, thyme, sage) to taste

1 kg potatoes, cut into cubes

Extra virgin olive oil

23 cloves garlic, minced

Juice of 1 lemon

Preparation:

Preheat the oven to 180°C. Season the pork roast with salt, pepper and herbs. on a baking tray, distribute the potato cubes evenly. Add the minced garlic, salt, pepper and a drizzle of olive oil. Mix well to cover the potatoes with the aromas. Place the pork roast on the baking sheet, on top of the potatoes. Squeeze lemon juice over the roast and add a drizzle of olive oil. Place the roasting pan in the preheated oven and cook for about 1 hour and 30 minutes, or until the roast reaches an internal temperature of at least 165°F and the potatoes are soft and golden. During cooking, check the roast and potatoes occasionally, turning the potatoes to make sure they cook evenly. Once cooked, remove the pork roast from the oven and let it rest for a few minutes before slicing. Serves the roast pork hot, accompanied by baked potatoes.

VENETIAN STYLE VEAL LIVER

Preparation times: approximately 10/15 minutes

Cooking times: approximately 20/25 minutes

Doses for 4 people

Ingredients:

500 g veal liver, cut into thin slices

Salt and pepper to taste Butter to taste

Flour to taste (to flour the liver)

23 medium onions, thinly sliced

1/2 cup white wine

Fresh parsley, chopped (optional)

Preparation:

Season the liver slices with salt and pepper and lightly flour both sides of the slices.

In a nonstick pan, melt some butter over medium-high heat. Add the liver slices to the pan and cook for 23 minutes per side, until well browned. Remove the liver from the pan and set aside. In the same pan, add another portion of butter if necessary and add the sliced onions. Cook the onions over medium-low heat until soft and lightly caramelized. Pour the white wine into the pan and let it evaporate for a few minutes. Add the browned liver slices to the pan with the onions and wine. Continue cooking the liver and onions together for another 57 minutes, or until the liver is cooked through but still soft in the center. Once ready, you can sprinkle the liver with a little chopped fresh parsley (optional). Serve the Venetian-style veal liver hot, accompanied by side dishes of your choice such as polenta, mashed potatoes or seasonal vegetables.

BEEF CHOP WITH TOMATO SAUCE

Preparation times: approximately 15/20 minutes

Cooking times: approximately 30/40 minutes

Doses for 4 people

Ingredients:

4 beef chops

Salt and Pepper To Taste

Flour to taste (to flour the chops)

Extra virgin olive oil

1 medium onion, finely chopped

23 cloves garlic, minced

400 g peeled tomatoes, chopped

1 teaspoon of sugar

Fresh basil, chopped (optional)

Preparation:

Season the beef chops with salt and pepper and lightly flour both sides. In a large skillet, heat some olive oil over medium-high heat. Add the chops to the pan and cook for 45 minutes per side, until well browned. Remove the chops from the pan and set aside. In the same pan, add a little olive oil if necessary and add the chopped onion. Cook the onion over medium-low heat until soft and translucent. Add the minced garlic to the pan with the onion and cook for another 12 minutes. Add the chopped peeled tomatoes to the pan with the onion and garlic. Also add the teaspoon of sugar to balance the acidity of the tomatoes.

Bring the tomato sauce to a boil, reduce the heat to medium-low and cook for about 15/20 minutes, or until the sauce thickens slightly. Add the beef chops to the tomato sauce and cook over medium-low heat for an additional 10/15 minutes, or until the chops are cooked through and tender. Before serving, you can sprinkle the chops with chopped fresh basil (optional).

PORK SAUSAGES WITH MASHED POTATOES

Preparation times: approximately 15/20 minutes

Cooking times: approximately 20/25 minutes

Doses for 4 people

Ingredients:

4 pork sausages

Extra virgin olive oil

4 medium potatoes, peeled and cut into cubes

Salt to taste Butter to taste

Milk to taste Black pepper to taste

Fresh parsley, chopped (optional)

Preparation:

In a skillet, heat some olive oil over medium-high heat. Add the pork sausages to the pan and cook for 10 to 12 minutes, turning occasionally, until well cooked and browned. Meanwhile, in a saucepan, bring lightly salted water to the boil and add the potato cubes. Cook the potatoes until tender, then drain. Mash the cooked potatoes with a pinch of salt, a little butter and a little milk. Continue mashing until you get a smooth, creamy consistency. Add black pepper to taste. Once ready, serve the hot pork sausages with the mashed potatoes.

BARBECUE LAMB RIBS

Preparation times: approximately 20 minutes

Cooking times: approximately 1 hour and 30 minutes

Doses for 4 people

Ingredients:

1 kg of lamb ribs

Salt and Pepper To Taste

Sweet paprika to taste

1/2 cup barbecue sauce

2 tablespoons soy sauce

2 tablespoons honey

Juice of 1 lemon

2 cloves garlic, finely chopped

Extra virgin olive oil

Preparation:

Preheat barbecue grill to medium-high heat. Season the lamb ribs with salt, pepper and sweet paprika. In a bowl, mix together the barbecue sauce, soy sauce, honey, lemon juice and minced garlic. Brush the lamb ribs with the prepared marinade, making sure to cover all sides well. Place the lamb ribs on the barbecue grill and cook for about 1 hour and 30 minutes, turning occasionally and brushing with the remaining marinade. While cooking, check that the ribs are cooked but still tender and juicy. Once ready, remove the lamb ribs from the barbecue and let them rest for a few minutes before serving. Serve the hot barbecue lamb ribs, accompanied by side dishes of your choice such as salad, baked potatoes or grilled vegetables.

GRILLED DUCK STEAK

Preparation times: approximately 15 minutes

Cooking times: approximately 10 minutes

Doses for 4 people

Ingredients:

4 duck steaks

Salt and Pepper To Taste

2 tablespoons extra virgin olive oil

2 cloves garlic, finely chopped

Fresh rosemary, chopped (optional)

Juice of 1 lemon

Preparation:

Preheat grill to medium-high heat. Season the duck steaks with salt, pepper and extra virgin olive oil. Add minced garlic and fresh rosemary to the meat, if desired. Place the duck steaks on the grill and cook for about 45 minutes per side, or until well browned on the outside and pink in the center. While cooking, brush the steaks with lemon juice to add a touch of freshness. Once cooked, remove the duck steaks from the grill and let them rest for a few minutes before serving. Serve the grilled duck steaks hot, accompanied by side dishes of your choice such as roast potatoes, grilled vegetables or mixed salad.

CHICKEN WITH LEMON AND PARSLEY

Preparation times: approximately 15 minutes

Cooking times: approximately 30/35 minutes

Doses for 4 people

Ingredients:

4 chicken breasts

Salt and Pepper To Taste

Juice of 2 lemons

Grated zest of 1 lemon

Fresh parsley, finely chopped

Extra virgin olive oil

Preparation:

Preheat the oven to 200°C. Season the chicken breasts with salt, pepper, lemon juice and grated lemon zest. Heat some olive oil in a pan over medium-high heat. Add the chicken breasts to the pan and cook for 23 minutes per side, until golden brown. Transfer the chicken breasts to a baking tray and cook in the preheated oven for approximately 25 to 30 minutes, or until fully cooked and juicy. During the last minutes of cooking, sprinkle the chicken breasts with chopped fresh parsley. Remove the lemon and parsley chicken from the oven and serve hot, accompanied by side dishes of your choice such as rice pilaf, roast potatoes or steamed vegetables.

PORK FILLET WRAPPED IN BACON

Preparation times: approximately 15 minutes

Cooking times: approximately 30 minutes

Doses for 4 people

Ingredients:

4 pork fillets

Salt and Pepper To Taste

8 slices of bacon

Extra virgin olive oil

Preparation:

Preheat the oven to 200°C. Season the pork tenderloins with salt and pepper. Wrap each pork tenderloin with 2 slices of bacon, making sure to cover the meat well. Heat some olive oil in a pan over medium-high heat. Add the bacon-wrapped pork tenderloins to the pan and cook for 23 minutes per side, until the bacon is crispy. Transfer the pork tenderloins to the baking sheet and bake in the preheated oven for about 25 minutes, or until cooked through and juicy. Remove the bacon-wrapped pork fillet from the oven and let it rest for a few minutes before serving. Serve the pork tenderloin hot, accompanied by side dishes of your choice such as baked potatoes, mashed potatoes or grilled vegetables.

PAN-FRIED CHICKEN LIVER

Preparation time: 10 minutes

Cooking times: 10 minutes

for 4 people:

Ingredients:

500 g of chicken liver

Salt to taste

Pepper as needed

Flour to taste

Olive oil to taste

1 medium onion,

sliced (optional)

Preparation:

Clean the chicken liver thoroughly, removing any fatty parts or unwanted ribs. Cut the chicken liver into thin slices and season with salt and pepper. Dredge the liver slices in the flour, shaking lightly to remove the excess. Heat some olive oil in a nonstick pan over medium-high heat. Add the chicken liver to the pan and cook for about 4/5 minutes per side, until golden and a light crust forms. If desired, add the onion slices to the pan and sauté them together with the liver for a couple of minutes. Serve the pan-fried chicken liver hot.

VENIS STEAK WITH BLUEBERRY SAUCE

Preparation times: 15/20 minutes

+ 10/15 minutes for the blueberry sauce

Cooking times: 4 to 8 minutes per side

for 4 people:

Ingredients

4 venison steak (about 200 g each)

Salt to taste Pepper to taste

Olive oil to taste

200 g of fresh or frozen blueberries

1/4 cup sugar

Juice of half a lemon

1/2 cup beef broth

Preparation:

Preheat the oven to 180°C. Season the venison steaks with salt and pepper. Heat a a little olive oil in a heatproof pan over medium-high heat. Add the venison steaks to the pan and cook for 24 minutes per side, depending on your desired doneness preference. Transfer the steaks to a baking tray and cook them in the preheated oven for a further 5/10 minutes, if necessary, to reach the desired doneness. In the meantime, prepare the blueberry sauce: in a saucepan, add the blueberries, sugar, lemon juice and meat broth or venison cooking juices. Bring to the boil and reduce the heat to medium-low. Cook for about 10/15 minutes, until the blueberries break down and the sauce thickens slightly. If the sauce is too liquid, you can add a teaspoon of corn starch dissolved in a little water to thicken it. Once done, let the steaks rest for a few minutes before slicing. Serve the venison steak slices with the hot cranberry sauce. You can add side dishes as desired, such as baked potatoes or grilled vegetables.

MEATBALLS WITH SAUCE

Preparation times: 20/30 minutes

Cooking times: 20/25 minutes

Preparation of the sauce: 15/20 minutes

for 4 people:

Ingredients

For the meatballs:

500 g minced meat (beef,

pork, veal or a combination)

1 egg, 1/2 cup breadcrumbs

1/4 cup shredded cheese

(Parmesan or Pecorino)

1 clove garlic, finely chopped

2 tablespoons chopped fresh parsley

Salt and pepper to taste. Olive oil to taste

For the sauce: 2 tablespoons of olive oil

1 medium onion, finely chopped

2 cloves garlic, finely chopped

1 can (400 g) peeled tomatoes

1/2 cup beef broth or water

Salt and Pepper To Taste

Fresh basil for garnish (optional)

Preparation:

For the meatballs: In a large bowl, combine the ground beef, egg, breadcrumbs, grated cheese, garlic, parsley, salt and pepper. Mix well until a homogeneous mixture is obtained. Form meatballs of the desired size with your hands, rounding and compacting slightly. Heat some olive oil in a nonstick pan over medium-high heat.

Add the meatballs to the pan and cook for about 10/12 minutes, turning them gently to brown them on all sides. Once cooked, transfer the meatballs to a plate and cover them with aluminum foil to keep them warm. For the sauce: In the same pan used for the meatballs, heat the olive oil over medium heat. Add the chopped onion and garlic and fry until soft and golden. Add the peeled tomatoes crushed with your hands and the meat broth. Mix well and bring the sauce to the boil. Reduce the heat to medium-low and let the sauce cook for about 10/15 minutes, until it thickens slightly. Season with salt and pepper to taste. Add the meatballs to the sauce and leave to cook for another 5 minutes, to let them flavor and heat through. Serve the meatballs with sauce hot, sprinkled with fresh basil (if desired).

PORK CHOPS
WITH MUSTARD

Preparation time: 15 minutes

Cooking times: 15/20 minutes

for 4 people:

Ingredients

8 pork chops

Salt and Pepper To Taste

2 tablespoons Dijon mustard

2 tablespoons honey

2 tablespoons of olive oil

Preparation:

Preheat the oven to 200°C. Season the pork chops with salt and pepper on both sides.

In a small bowl, mix the Dijon mustard and honey until smooth. Spread the honey-mustard sauce on both sides of the pork chops. Heat the olive oil in a heatproof skillet over medium-high heat. Add the ribs to the pan and cook them for about 3/4 minutes per side, until a golden crust forms. Transfer the ribs to a baking tray and cook them in the preheated oven for a further 10 to 12 minutes, or until cooked to the desired point. Once cooked, let the ribs rest for a few minutes before serving. Serve the mustard pork chops hot, accompanied by side dishes of your choice, such as baked potatoes or grilled vegetables.

BEEF STEAK WITH
GARLIC BUTTER

Preparation times: 10/15 minutes

Cooking times: 4 to 8 minutes per side

for 4 people:

Ingredients:

4 beef steaks (about 200 g each)

Salt and Pepper To Taste

Olive oil to taste

4 tablespoons butter

4 cloves garlic, finely chopped

Chopped fresh parsley for garnish (optional)

Preparation:

Preheat the oven to 180°C. Season the beef steaks with salt and pepper on both sides. Heat some olive oil in a heatproof pan over medium-high heat. Add the steaks to the pan and cook for 24 minutes per side, depending on your desired doneness preference. Transfer the steaks to a baking tray and cook them in the preheated oven for a further 5/10 minutes, if necessary, to reach the desired doneness. Meanwhile, in a small skillet, melt the butter over medium-low heat. Add the minced garlic and fry for about 12 minutes, until golden and fragrant. Once cooked, let the steaks rest for a few minutes before serving. Pour the garlic butter over the steaks just before serving and garnish with chopped fresh parsley (if desired).

CHICKEN CURRY

Preparation times: 15/20 minutes

Cooking times: 25/30 minutes

for 4 people:

Ingredients:

4 chicken breasts, cut into cubes

Salt and Pepper To Taste

2 tablespoons vegetable oil

1 medium onion, finely chopped

2 cloves garlic, finely chopped

2 tablespoons curry powder

1 can (400ml) coconut milk

1 cup chicken broth

2 carrots, cut into thin slices

1 bell pepper, cut into cubes

Preparation:

Season the chicken cubes with salt and pepper. Heat vegetable oil in a skillet over medium-high heat. Add the chicken to the pan and cook until golden brown on all sides. Remove the chicken from the pan and set aside. In the same pan, add the chopped onion and garlic. Fry them until they become soft and golden. Add the curry powder and mix well for 12 minutes to release the flavours. Add coconut milk and chicken broth. Mix well and bring everything to the boil. Reduce the heat to medium-low and add the carrots and bell pepper. Cover the pan and cook for about 15/20 minutes, or until the vegetables are tender. Add the chicken cubes to the pan and cook for a further 5 to 10 minutes, until the chicken is cooked through and the sauce thickens slightly. Once ready, serve the chicken curry hot, accompanied by basmati rice or naan.

PORK CHOPS WITH PORCINI MUSHROOM SAUCE

Preparation times: 15/20 minutes

Cooking times: 12/15 minutes

for 4 people:

Ingredients:

4 pork chops, about 150g each

Salt and Pepper To Taste

2 tablespoons of olive oil

1 medium onion, finely chopped

200 g of fresh porcini mushrooms

or dried (soaked and wrung out)

1 cup beef broth

1/2 cup heavy cream

Preparation:

Season the pork chops with salt and pepper on both sides. Heat the olive oil in a skillet over medium-high heat. Add the pork chops to the pan and cook for about 6 to 8 minutes per side, until cooked through and golden brown. Remove the chops from the pan and keep warm. In the same pan, add the chopped onion and porcini mushrooms. Cook them until the onion becomes soft and the mushrooms are golden. Add the beef broth to the pan and bring everything to a boil. Reduce the heat to medium-low and leave to cook for about 58 minutes, until the sauce thickens slightly. Add the cooking cream to the pan and mix well. Continue to cook for another 23 minutes, until the sauce is well blended and creamy. Once ready, serve the pork chops hot, accompanied by the porcini mushroom sauce.

TURKEY SAUSAGES WITH

ROASTED PEPPERS

Preparation time: 20 minutes

Cooking times: 30/40 minutes

for 4 people:

Ingredients :

8 turkey sausages

2 tablespoons of olive oil

2 peppers of different colors,

cut into strips

Salt and Pepper To Taste

Chopped fresh parsley

for garnish (optional)

Preparation:

Preheat the oven to 200°C. Arrange the strips of peppers on a baking tray and season with salt, pepper and a drizzle of olive oil. Mix well to coat the peppers. Cook the peppers in the preheated oven for about 20/25 minutes, until they are soft and lightly golden. Remove them from the oven and keep them aside. Meanwhile, heat the olive oil in a skillet over medium-high heat. Add the turkey sausages to the pan and cook for about 5 to 6 minutes per side, until cooked through and golden brown. Once ready, serve the turkey sausages hot, accompanied by the roasted peppers. Garnish with chopped fresh parsley (if desired).

VEAL STEAK WITH
RED WINE SAUCE

Preparation time: 20 minutes

Cooking times: 35 minutes per side)

for 4 people:

Ingredients:

4 veal steaks (about 200 g each)

Salt and pepper to taste, Olive oil to taste

1 medium onion, finely chopped

2 cloves garlic, finely chopped

200 ml of red wine,

200 ml of meat broth

2 tablespoons cold butter,

cut into cubes

Preparation:

Season the veal steaks with salt and pepper on both sides. Heat some olive oil in a pan over medium-high heat. Add the steaks to the pan and cook for 35 minutes per side, depending on your desired doneness preference. Remove steaks from pan and keep warm. In the same pan, add the chopped onion and garlic. Fry them until they become soft and golden. Add the red wine to the pan and let it reduce by about half over medium-high heat. Add the beef broth to the pan and bring everything to a boil. Reduce the heat to medium-low and leave to cook for about 5/8 minutes, until the sauce thickens slightly. Remove the pan from the heat and add the cold cubed butter. Mix well until the butter melts and the sauce becomes creamy. Once ready, serve the veal steaks hot, accompanied by the red wine sauce.

CHILLI CHICKEN

Preparation time: 20 minutes

Cooking times: 20/25 minutes

for 4 people:

Ingredients:

4 chicken breasts, skinless and boneless

Salt and Pepper To Taste

2 tablespoons of olive oil

34 fresh red chillies, cut into rounds

3 cloves garlic, finely chopped

Juice of 1 lemon

Preparation:

Season the chicken breasts with salt and pepper on both sides. Heat the olive oil in a skillet over medium-high heat. Add the chicken to the pan and cook for about 10/12 minutes per side, until well cooked and golden. Remove the chicken from the pan and keep warm. In the same pan, add the red chilies and minced garlic. Fry them for 12 minutes, until they become soft and fragrant. Add the lemon juice to the pan and mix well. Put the chicken back in the pan and cook it together with the chillies and garlic for another 23 minutes, so that they flavor well. Once ready, serve the chilli chicken hot.

LAMB IN AROMATIC HERBS CRUST

Preparation time: 25 minutes

Cooking times: 30 minutes

for 4 people:

Ingredients:

4 lamb chops

Salt and Pepper To Taste

2 tablespoons Dijon mustard

2 cloves garlic, finely chopped

2 tablespoons fresh parsley, chopped

1 tablespoon fresh thyme, chopped

1 tablespoon fresh rosemary, chopped

2 tablespoons of breadcrumbs

2 tablespoons of olive oil

Preparation:

Preheat the oven to 200°C. Salt and pepper the lamb chops on both sides. In a bowl, mix the Dijon mustard, minced garlic, parsley, thyme and rosemary. Spread the herb mixture evenly over the surface of the lamb chops. Sprinkle breadcrumbs over the chops to create a crust. Heat the olive oil in a heatproof pan and brown the lamb chops on both sides until a golden crust forms. Transfer the lamb chops to the baking tray and cook in the preheated oven for 25 to 30 minutes, or until the lamb reaches the desired doneness. Serve the lamb chops encrusted with hot aromatic herbs.

BREADED CHICKEN CUTLET

Preparation time: 15 minutes

Cooking times: 10/12 minutes

for 4 people:

Ingredients:

4 chicken breasts

Salt and Pepper To Taste

Flour to taste

2 eggs, beaten

Breadcrumbs to taste

Olive oil for frying

Preparation:

Set up a breading station with three separate bowls: one with flour, one with beaten eggs, and one with breadcrumbs. Salt and pepper the chicken breasts on both sides. Dip each chicken breast in the flour, then in the beaten egg and finally in the breadcrumbs, pressing lightly to make the breadcrumbs stick. Heat plenty of olive oil in a pan over medium-high heat. Fry the breaded chicken cutlets in the pan, turning once, until golden brown and crispy on both sides, about 5 to 6 minutes per side. Drain the cutlets on absorbent paper to remove excess oil. Serve the breaded chicken cutlets hot with side dishes of your choice.

BEEF STEAK WITH BLUEBERRY SAUCE

Preparation time: 10 minutes

Cooking times: 10/12 minutes

for 4 people:

Ingredients:

4 beef steak

(approximately 200/250 g each)

Salt and Pepper To Taste

Olive oil for cooking

1 cup fresh or frozen blueberries

2 tablespoons of sugar, Juice of 1/2 lemon

1/2 cup beef broth

1 tablespoon cornflour (corn starch)

diluted in 2 tablespoons of cold water

Preparation:

R Heat a non-stick pan over medium-high heat. Salt and pepper the beef steaks on both sides. Add a drizzle of olive oil to the pan and place the steaks. Cook steaks for 46 minutes per side, depending on thickness and desired doneness. Remove the steaks from the pan and let them rest on a foil-covered plate for a few minutes. Meanwhile, in the same pan, add the blueberries, sugar, lemon juice and beef broth. Bring to the boil. Reduce the heat and simmer for about 5 minutes until the blueberries break down and the sauce begins to thicken slightly. Gradually add the cornstarch diluted in the cold water, stirring constantly until the sauce thickens further. Serve the beef steaks with the hot cranberry sauce.

STUFFED MEATLOAF

Preparation time: 20 minutes

Cooking Times: 45/50 minutes

for 4 people:

Ingredients:

500g of minced meat

(beef, pork or mixed)

100 g of breadcrumbs

1/4 cup milk

100 g of grated cheese

(Parmesan or Pecorino)

2 cloves garlic, finely chopped

2 tablespoons fresh parsley, chopped

Salt and pepper to taste 1 egg

Sliced cheese

(mozzarella or provola)

1/2 cup tomato sauce

(or marinara sauce)

Preparation:

Preheat the oven to 180°C. In a bowl, mix the ground beef, egg, breadcrumbs, milk, grated cheese, garlic, parsley, salt and pepper until smooth. Prepare a rectangular shape of meat on the work surface. Arrange the cheese slices in the center of the meat rectangle. Roll the meat on itself, sealing the edges well to form a stuffed meatloaf.

Transfer the meatloaf to a lightly oiled baking pan. Pour the tomato sauce over the meatloaf. Cook in the preheated oven for 45/50 minutes or until the meatloaf is well cooked and golden. Let it rest for a few minutes before slicing the meatloaf. Serve the stuffed meatloaf with the hot tomato sauce.

PORK STEAK WITH APPLE SAUCE

Preparation time: 10 minutes

Cooking times: 12/15 minutes

for 4 people:

Ingredients:

4 pork steaks (200 g each)

Salt and Pepper To Taste

Olive oil for cooking

2 green apples, peeled

and cut into thin slices

2 tablespoons butter

1/4 cup chicken broth

1/4 cup heavy cream

1 tablespoon Dijon mustard

1 tablespoon of sugar

Preparation:

R Heat a non-stick pan over medium-high heat. Salt and pepper the pork steaks on both sides. Add a drizzle of olive oil to the pan and place the steaks. Cook the steaks for 6 to 8 minutes per side, or until cooked through and golden brown. Remove the steaks from the pan and let them rest on a plate covered with foil. In the same pan, add the butter and apple slices. Cook the apples until soft and lightly browned. Add the chicken broth, heavy cream, Dijon mustard and sugar. Mix well and bring to the boil. Reduce the heat and let simmer for about 5 minutes, until the sauce thickens slightly. Serve pork steaks with hot applesauce.

SHRIMP AND BACON SKEWERS

Preparation time: 15 minutes

Cooking times: Grilled: 68 minutes

for 4 people:

Ingredients:

16 large prawns, peeled

and deprived of the black filament

8 slices of smoked bacon, cut in half

Juice of 1 lemon

2 tablespoons of olive oil

Salt and Pepper To Taste

1 teaspoon sweet paprika (optional)

Fresh rosemary sprigs (optional, for garnish)

Preparation:

Preheat grill to medium-high heat. In a bowl, combine the lemon juice, olive oil, salt, pepper, and sweet paprika (if desired). Thread a shrimp onto a piece of bacon and fold the bacon around the shrimp. Repeat with the remaining shrimp and bacon slices. Brush the skewers with the lemon and olive oil marinade. Place the shrimp skewers on the grill and cook for 34 minutes per side, turning once, until the bacon is crisp and the shrimp are cooked through. Serve the shrimp and bacon skewers hot, garnished with sprigs of fresh rosemary, if desired.

DUCK STEAK WITH ORANGE SAUCE

Preparation time: 10 minutes

Cooking times: 10/12 minutes

for 4 people:

Ingredients:

4 duck steak

(approximately 250 g each)

Salt and Pepper To Taste

Olive oil for cooking

2 oranges, juice and grated zest

2 tablespoons honey

2 tablespoons red wine vinegar

1/2 cup chicken broth

1 tablespoon cornflour (corn starch)

diluted in 2 tablespoons of cold water

Preparation:

R Heat a non-stick pan over medium-high heat. Salt and pepper the duck steaks on both sides. Add a drizzle of olive oil to the pan and place the steaks. Cook steaks for 46 minutes per side, depending on thickness and desired doneness. Remove the steaks from the pan and let them rest on a foil-covered plate for a few minutes. In the same pan, add the juice and grated zest of the oranges, honey, red wine vinegar and chicken broth. Bring to the boil. Reduce the heat and let simmer for about 5 minutes to thicken the sauce slightly. Gradually add the cornstarch diluted in the cold water, stirring constantly until the sauce thickens further. Serve the duck steaks with the hot orange sauce.

CHICKEN WITH ROSEMARY AND LEMON

Preparation time: 10 minutes

Cooking times: 15/20 minutes

for 4 people:

Ingredients:

4 chicken breasts

Salt and Pepper To Taste

Juice of 2 lemons

Grated zest of 1 lemon

2 tablespoons of olive oil

2 cloves garlic, finely chopped

23 sprigs of fresh rosemary

1/2 cup chicken broth

Preparation:

In a bowl, mix the lemon juice, grated lemon zest, olive oil, minced garlic, salt and pepper. If you wish, you can marinate the chicken breasts in the lemon and olive oil mixture for about 30 minutes. R Heat a non-stick pan over medium-high heat. Remove the chicken breasts from the marinade (if you marinated) and pat dry lightly with paper towels. Add the chicken breasts to the skillet and cook for 68 minutes per side, until browned and cooked through. Add the rosemary sprigs and chicken broth to the pan. Cover with a lid and continue to cook for another 57 minutes, or until the chicken is fully cooked and the broth has reduced slightly. Remove the chicken breasts from the pan and let them rest for a few minutes before serving. You can serve the rosemary and lemon chicken with side dishes of your choice.

CONCLUSION

Thank you for taking the time to explore "Carnivore Diet 2025." I hope the information, practical advice and recipes included have inspired and guided you on your journey to better health and optimal well-being. Adopting a carnivore diet can be a powerful and transformative choice, and your commitment is the first step towards real, lasting results. If you found the book useful and interesting, I would be grateful if you could share your experience by leaving a review. Your words not only help other readers discover the book, but they also provide valuable feedback that helps me improve and offer even more useful content in the future. Thanks again for your time and support. I wish you a fruitful and satisfying nutritional journey!

[KLARLOCK]